Chair Yoga for Seniors to Lose Weight

Easy Seated Exercises to Shed Belly Fat, Regain Mobility and Flexibility in Just 10 Minutes a Day

By Michael Smith

Copyright © Michael Smith - All rights reserved.

The content contained within this book may not be reproduced, duplicated or transmitted without direct written permission from the author or the publisher.

Under no circumstances will any blame or legal responsibility be held against the publisher, or author, for any damages, reparation, or monetary loss due to the information contained within this book. Either directly or indirectly. You are responsible for your own choices, actions, and results.

Legal Notice:

This book is copyright protected. This book is only for personal use. You cannot amend, distribute, sell, use, quote or paraphrase any part, or the content within this book, without the consent of the author or publisher.

Disclaimer Notice:

Please note the information contained within this document is for educational and entertainment purposes only. All effort has been executed to present accurate, up to date, and reliable, complete information. No warranties of any kind are declared or implied. Readers acknowledge that the author is not engaging in the rendering of legal, financial, medical or professional advice. The content within this book has been derived from various sources. Please consult a licensed professional before attempting any techniques outlined in this book.

By reading this document, the reader agrees that under no circumstances is the author responsible for any losses, direct or indirect, which are incurred as a result of the use of the information contained within this document, including, but not limited to, — errors, omissions, or inaccuracies.

TABLE OF CONTENTS

INTRODUCTION 1

CHAPTER 1: Why Chair Yoga for Seniors? 5

CHAPTER 2: Getting Started with Chair Yoga 10
- Cat cow pose 20
- Wrist rotation 22
- Toe rotations 22
- Shoulder circles 23
- Pelvic tilt 23
- Neck stretches 24

CHAPTER 3: 18 Simple but Effective Chair Yoga Poses 26
- Poses for mobility and flexibility 26
  - Seated Mountain Pose 28
  - Seated Forward Bend 29
  - Seated Butterfly Stretch 30
  - Seated Pigeon Pose 31
- Poses to strengthen the core 32
  - Seated Side Stretch 33
  - Seated Leg Lifts 34
  - Seated Boat Pose 35
  - Seated Bicycle Crunches 36
- Poses for better balance 37
  - Seated Tree Pose 37
  - Seated Chair Twist 38
  - Seated Warrior I 39
  - Chair Side Leg Lifts 40
- Poses to improve metabolism and digestion 41
  - Seated High Knee March 41
  - Seated Diaphragmatic Breathing 42
  - Chair High Lunge 43
  - Chair Downward Dog 46

    Child's Pose 49

    Cobra Pose 51

CHAPTER 4: 28-Day Challenge to Keep You Motivated 55

    FIRST WEEK 57

    SECOND WEEK 60

    THIRD WEEK 62

    FOURTH WEEK 64

CHAPTER 5: 10 Best Seated Exercises to Supercharge Your Weight Loss 67

    Seated Jumping Jacks 68

    Seated Toe Taps 70

    Seated Knee to Elbow 72

    Seated Cat-Cow Stretch - dynamic version 77

    Seated Shoulder Shrug 79

    Seated Leg Circles 81

    Reverse Crunches 82

    Seated Knee Head 83

    Seated Mountain Climbers 84

    Seated Mindful Breathing 85

CHAPTER 6: Chair Yoga in Under 10 Minutes 87

    Workout #1 - Beginner (and intermediate) level 89

    Workout #2 - Advanced level 96

CHAPTER 7: Chair Yoga Beyond Exercises: Stress Reduction and Mindful Eating 104

CONCLUSION 113

REFERENCES 116

INTRODUCTION

"It's going to be a journey. It's not a sprint to get in shape."
- **Kerri Walsh Jennings**

If you're looking for a workout that's appropriate for your age, I can confidently state that chair yoga is the safest and right choice. The reason for this is simple: **chair yoga is a low-intensity workout.**

Thanks to a consistent chair yoga practice, you will maintain your health and perform your daily activities with ease and a smile. The chair yoga exercises in this book will help you:

- Regain mobility and flexibility.
- Reduce pain in your ankles, wrists, neck, shoulders, back, and hips.
- Lose weight and move closer to your ideal weight.
- Establish a mindfulness lifestyle (proper breathing, proper eating).

Because chair yoga is a low-intensity workout, it is also ideal for those who have never exercised before.

As a personal trainer with experience working with clients of different ages, I have had the opportunity to gain insights into the reasons why people over 60 are more likely to gain weight.

Weight gain is not just about diet, especially for people over 60; diet is only one of the factors.

For years, I have had the honor of working with several clients who are over 70 years old, and by their energy and liveliness, I can easily compare them with clients who are two or three decades younger.

My clients who are 70+ years old boast excellent mobility and flexibility. Their body weight and muscle tone are at a very enviable level.

I even have a married couple, both 75 years old, who regularly compete in senior bike races. If you have ever ridden a bicycle, you are aware of how much mobility is required to maintain safety and prevent falls.

They were able to achieve all this thanks to the simple chair yoga exercises found inside this book.

They are grateful for the work I do, and I am very proud of them.

Why do we gain weight as we age?

As we age, various factors impact our weight; listed below are eight factors. However, keep in mind that to achieve your ideal body weight, it is paramount to address all the factors.

1. **Slowed Metabolism:** As you age, your metabolism slows down, causing your body to burn fewer calories at rest. Digestion slows down, and the absorption of nutrients reduces. However, most people do not consider this and continue to eat the same way they did when they were younger.

They consume the same number of calories or eat more due to reduced food absorption.

2. **Loss of muscle mass:** Muscular atrophy is a natural process associated with ageing. Although when it starts can vary, sarcopenia, an age-related decrease in muscle mass and strength, usually first appears in people around the age of 40. After hitting this milestone, adults may lose 3-5 percent of their muscle mass on average every ten years. Maintaining muscular health and reducing the consequences of sarcopenia require regular resistance training and a sufficient protein diet.

3. **Hormonal fluctuations**: Hormonal changes in women (postmenopausal) and men can lead to changes in metabolic functioning and fat distribution, causing weight gain.

4. **Physical activity:** Due to physical limitations, certain chronic conditions, or pain in the joints, people over 60 generally become less physically active.

Reduced physical activity and a sedentary lifestyle are well-known contributors of weight gain.

5. **Socialization:** Seniors (60+) become more isolated, are more susceptible to stress and depression, and therefore can resort to emotional eating.

With emotional eating, higher calories are consumed to fill an emotional void. This eating habit can quickly lead to weight gain.

6. **Health condition:** Many seniors (60+) who face certain chronic conditions also experience increased body weight.

Arthritis, diabetes, and mobility problems are some conditions that can lead to weight gain.

7. **Sleep:** Poor sleeping habits or sleep quality has an impact on appetite and can potentially lead to obesity.

8. **Medications:** Certain medications (prescribed or otherwise) can also lead to weight gain due to water retention or slowed metabolism.

You can do it too

If you manage to address these factors, you will attain the ideal weight for your age and physical constitution.

If you have gained weight because of certain medications, I recommend consulting your doctor to see if you can change your current therapy.

Although all eight factors are important, I believe physical exercise is more crucial.

Why?

Regular and appropriate physical activity is necessary to achieve the required mobility and flexibility. It also facilitates higher calorie burn, resulting in weight loss.

Trust me!

In this book, you will discover:

1. Why chair yoga is an excellent weight loss tool for people of all ages
2. The common misconceptions about yoga
3. How to start your **chair yoga practice simply** (necessary equipment, breathing techniques, and warming up the body)
4. 18 simple yet effective yoga positions for improving your mobility, flexibility, balance, metabolism, and digestion.
5. 10 most effective chair yoga positions for weight loss
6. Short yoga routines that will take less than 10 minutes to complete
7. How to implement chair yoga in your daily lifestyle (stress relief, mindful eating) **and much more...**

In the first chapter, we will explore why chair yoga is the best fitness solution for people of any age, the benefits of chair yoga, and the common misconceptions regarding yoga.

I will also show you how chair yoga can become your go-to weight loss tool.

The first chapter is awaiting us!

****

FREE GIFT #1: FULL AUDIO-BOOK

Did you know that listening to an audiobook can help you retain more information? Enjoy the audiobook anywhere, without needing to carry a physical book. By listening, you can engage in physical activities at the same time, giving your eyes a rest from reading.

To give it a try, visit **bit.ly/YogaBonuses** and grab the audio version (along with other free bonuses).

You can also scan the QR code with your phone camera if you prefer not to type. It's absolutely free.

I hope you find it helpful and enjoyable.

****

CHAPTER 1:
Why Chair Yoga for Seniors?

"An ounce of prevention is worth a pound of cure."

– Benjamin Franklin

What makes chair yoga a great fitness choice for seniors?

Chair yoga is an excellent choice for seniors to engage in physical activity, primarily for safety reasons. The exercises are performed while sitting on a chair or using a chair for support.

The chair yoga poses explored in this book have been modified and adapted for seniors.

Why chair yoga is an excellent choice for seniors:

Accessibility: There is no need to get down on the floor while practicing chair yoga. This is especially important for people who have limited mobility and flexibility.

Flexibility and Mobility: The poses performed while practicing chair yoga are not challenging and involve fine stretching, which is very important for seniors, especially those with limited flexibility and mobility.

Posture: Thanks to the chair yoga exercises and workouts in this book, you will improve your posture and thus reduce the possible risks of musculoskeletal problems.

Weight Loss: Practicing chair yoga poses designed for weight loss will help you achieve your ideal weight and tone your muscles.

Balance and Strength: With regular chair yoga practice, you will improve your sense of balance. You will also become stronger, minimizing the fear of possible falls due to balance issues or muscular weakness.

Pain Control: The very gentle stretching and rotation movements practiced in chair yoga can greatly reduce your eventual chronic pain.

Stress Control: By applying certain breathing and relaxation techniques, you will be able to improve your emotional and mental well-being.

Establishing a regular chair yoga practice is a great way to start your weight loss journey. Consistently practicing chair yoga helps improve metabolic functioning, sleep quality, flexibility and mobility, balance and strength, stress management, and nutrition.

Your physical and mental wellbeing will improve; you will develop healthier habits; and you will have a more positive outlook on life.

It is necessary to consult with a personal doctor and take precautionary measures

Consult your personal doctor before starting your chair yoga practice, especially if you have certain physical limitations or any concerns.

Preferably, show your doctor the exercises you plan to practice.

If you have certain breathing problems, explore the breathing techniques with your doctor so you can ensure that the breathing techniques are safe for you.

Do not force your body during the exercises. Respect the current limitations of your body to avoid pain and discomfort.

Chair yoga as an effective tool for weight loss

Chair yoga can be an effective weight-loss tool, but don't expect dramatic results overnight.

Practicing chair yoga will impact various physical and psychological factors that influence body weight.

- When you are under stress, you generally calm your nervous system by eating high calorie foods.

  Such food is called emotional food.

  With regular chair yoga practice, you will no longer need emotional food and will be able to control your stress level.

- By practicing the mindfulness techniques found in this book, you will begin to eat more consciously, aware of your every bite.

  You will no longer eat in a hurry; you will take enough time for each of your meals. You will develop healthier eating habits, contributing to weight loss.

- Although it is a low-impact physical activity, chair yoga can boost your metabolism. This will result in a better and faster expenditure of calories, facilitating weight loss.
- The breathing techniques incorporated in chair yoga practice will improve the quality of your sleep. Keep in mind that poor sleep contributes to weight gain.
- Regular chair yoga practice will improve your mobility, which leads to more calories burned, fueling weight loss.
- Chair yoga practice is ideal for seniors because it offers a gentle, accessible practice that can be tailored to different mobility levels, it's a great option for seniors. For those with a limited range of motion or balance problems, using a chair adds stability and added support, increasing safety. This style of yoga helps to improve general well-being by fostering strength, flexibility, and relaxation without placing undue strain on aging joints.
- By practicing chair yoga, the support provided by the chair reduces the risk of injury.

In the long term, chair yoga is an effective weight loss strategy, especially when viewed from a holistic point of view.

Seven myths and misconceptions about yoga

Yoga is a discipline that is more than 5000 years old, offering a variety of benefits (physical, mental, and spiritual), including achieving ideal body weight.

Yoga has been subject to misconceptions in the West for decades, with some of them including:

1. **Yoga is only for women** - This is one of the biggest misconceptions, considering that the first yogis (people who practice yoga) were men. Most yoga postures were designed for the male body. Over time, poses have been modified and new poses created that are in harmony with the female body.

   This misconception has permeated because globally, more women practice yoga. However, this has changed over time as yoga has become an integral part of training for professional athletes.

   As a result, men are beginning to accept yoga as an integral part of their physical training.

2. **Yoga is a religion** - Yoga itself is not religious, although it has roots in various philosophical and spiritual traditions.

   You can practice yoga without accepting any belief system. This is especially true in the West, where yoga classes emphasize the physical and mental aspects of yoga.

3. **Yoga is practiced by the flexible** - You practice yoga to improve your flexibility. In yoga, the most important thing is making progress, not how you were at the beginning of your practice.

4. **Yoga is easy; it only involves relaxation** - As a discipline, yoga has over 100 different styles, with some being more physically demanding than others.

   Vinyasa and Ashtanga yoga, for example, are very physically demanding systems, while Yin yoga is very gentle and peaceful.

5. **Equipment is expensive** - Basic yoga equipment is inexpensive, and this applies to chair yoga as well. With chair yoga, all you need is a sturdy chair and comfortable clothes.

   All other equipment is optional.

6. **Yoga is for the young** - The truth is, yoga is for all ages. The beauty of yoga is that all poses can be easily adapted to different psychophysical abilities.

7. **Yoga is purely a physical discipline** - Yoga postures are an important part of yoga as a discipline, but they represent only one aspect.

   If you want to master different breathing, meditation, and relaxation techniques, yoga can help. Yoga is a discipline that deals with your body, mind, and spirit.

In the first chapter, you learned why chair yoga is a good physical activity for seniors. You have discovered how chair yoga practice can help you in your pursuit of your ideal weight. You were introduced to the benefits of yoga and the facts that showed you how chair yoga can be an effective tool for weight loss.

You've explored the seven biggest yoga myths and misconceptions.

I believe you are eager to get going. In the second chapter, we will explore how to start your chair yoga practice.

You will discover what you need for your practice (a suitable chair, space, and atmosphere), why breathing is so important in yoga, and the basic breathing techniques.

You will learn how to be mindful in every moment, how to protect your body, and warm up properly.

CHAPTER 2:
Getting Started with Chair Yoga

"Things change, so I have to change too."

- Adam Scythe

How to reorganize your way of thinking

Every beginning brings challenges. When you start new projects, you have to "reorganize" your way of thinking, especially if you had no experience in that field before.

In every beginning, it is difficult to remain consistent and constant.

This is also true when starting your chair yoga practice. Before starting your chair yoga practice, it is very important to create a positive attitude that you will incorporate into your daily activities.

To create a positive attitude and achieve mindfulness during your chair yoga practice, I advise you to start with the following daily mini practices:

- **Gratitude -** Start being thankful for everything in your life. When you are grateful, you raise the frequency of your being, which positively affects your way of thinking and your overall health.

  The more positive you are, obstacles become challenges you can overcome.

  The easiest way to start this mini practice is to have some kind of trigger that will remind you to be grateful.

  For example, you can put a small stone in your pocket, and whenever you touch it, it can be your trigger. At that moment, give thanks for whatever comes to mind (green grass, the sun shining, the conversation you just had...)

- **Surround yourself with positive people -** I believe you are familiar with the proverb, "You are who you are with!"

It is believed that you are essentially a reflection of the five people you are most in contact with. Think about the five people you hang out with the most.

If you conclude that certain people are not good influences, feel free to change your environment. Find new people in different social circles (you can start volunteering and help other people that way).

Surround yourself with people with good energy—people who are positive. Such people will inspire you; they will be the initiators of your new ideas and projects.

The social interaction you have with the people in your immediate environment greatly affects your way of thinking and your attitudes.

- **Smile and sing more** - Your brain cannot distinguish reality from imagination. That is why it is not difficult to always have a smile on your face.

Laughing also raises the frequency of your being.

As for singing, if you believe you don't have a singing voice, there is a solution for that. Sing while showering or relaxing in the tub.

Let your voice free you from all the accumulated negativity and fill you with positivity. Just remember the proverb: "He who sings does not think evil!"

- **Don't let anything upset you** - When a situation happens to derail you, ask yourself two questions: "Will this matter to me in a week, a year, or 5 years? Will I not be able to continue with my life because of this?"

You will see that everything is solvable and that there is nothing that should eat you up inside. You don't need to be constantly exposed to stress for any reason.

Just remember the Tibetan proverb: "If you can change the situation, there is no need to be upset. If you can't change the situation, there's no need to get upset."

- **See obstacles as challenges** - Don't allow yourself to be held back or limited by anything in life.

This way, you will never put things off again, but you will tackle the problem right away because you will no longer see the problem as an obstacle but as a challenge.

- **Write a journal** - Write down your thoughts, emotions, and life events. You can do that in the form of prose, but also in the form of poetry.

  Let the sentences "write themselves." Don't think too much about the writing style. The first thing you write in your journal represents your truth, honest feelings, and thoughts.

It's best to start these mini practices a week or two before starting your chair yoga practice. During this period, you will be able to "reorganize" your way of thinking.

If you are unable to practice all the above mini practices, it is perfectly fine to start with one. You can add others over time.

TIP: Make mini practices an integral part of your daily activities, not just a part of the chair yoga practice. In this way, you will succeed in creating a new lifestyle filled with positivity and mindfulness.

Thanks to these mini practices, your chair yoga practice will be more mindful.

Equipment and space for a safe and successful chair yoga practice

Once you reorganize your mindset, you can embark on securing the necessary space and equipment for your chair yoga practice.

For chair yoga, the necessary equipment includes a chair, appropriate clothing, shoes, and a yoga mat.

Appropriate equipment will allow you to safely practice chair yoga, allowing you to enter certain positions more easily.

By using the right equipment, you will prevent possible injuries.

- Yoga mat: When you decide on a yoga mat, ensure it is firm and thick enough. The yoga mat should provide the necessary stability for your feet and body.

- Clothing and shoes: The appropriate clothes and shoes will allow you move freely and exercise without any obstacles.

- Chair: A suitable chair will give you with the necessary support and stability during your chair yoga practice. Keep in mind that the chair must not rock when you sit or stand on it.

Ensure that, while sitting in the chair, your knees remain above your ankles. Don't buy a chair with wheels; a chair with legs is a must for your chair yoga practice to provide the necessary stability and firmness.

When purchasing the necessary equipment, follow your personal preferences; however, comfort and quality materials should also influence your equipment selection.

You do not need a large financial investment to get the necessary equipment for chair yoga practice, especially since most of the equipment is already in your home.

When deciding on the space to practice chair yoga, it is important to pay attention to the following factors:

- The space should be of suitable size. This means that there is enough room for your chair, you, and your movement during the exercise.

  The easiest way to determine if the space is the right size is to ensure that you have enough space to comfortably walk around the chair.

  To determine if there is enough room for movement during the exercise, stand in the middle of the room, raise your hands to shoulder height, and turn in a full circle. If you do not touch the walls of the room with your fingers, the space is suitable.

- It is recommended to have at least one window in the room you choose to practice chair yoga. This will ensure a constant flow of fresh air.

- The space in which you practice should be empty; remove any carpets in the room and place your chair on a yoga mat. It is much firmer than most carpets.

- Play spa or meditative music in the background if you want to create a relaxed atmosphere during exercise. You can also use various scented oils or incense sticks.

Basic breathing techniques and mindfulness

Thanks to breathing, your organs and body work in harmony. Although breathing is an involuntary activity (it happens even if you don't pay attention to it), you can become aware of your breathing and thus turn breathing into a voluntary activity.

When you start applying the basic breathing techniques described in this chapter, your life will change radically, especially if you realize that you are currently breathing in an uneven rhythm (short inhalations and exhalations that are very often interrupted).

By becoming aware of your breathing:
- You will be more present in the moment.
- Your focus and concentration will be significantly better.
- You will be fully aware of your movement both during your chair yoga practice and the rest of the day.
- Your body will relax better and faster.
- Oxygen supply to your cells and organs will improve.

By incorporating basic breathing techniques into your chair yoga practice and daily routine, you will notice a great improvement in your mobility and flexibility.

Three-layer breathing

During each breath, it is important that your back is completely straight and supported by the back of the chair.

Three-layer breathing means that you breathe in segments through the nose (the stomach, lungs, and tops of the lungs). By applying three-layer breathing, you will supply every part of your body with the necessary oxygen. With three-layer breathing, you will get rid of accumulated stagnant air from the lower part of the stomach.

While practicing chair yoga, you will always use this breathing technique, while the other breathing techniques can be applied before or after your practice.

Belly breathing - To become fully aware of belly breathing, place both palms on your belly. Do not forget that your back must be completely straight and supported by the back of the chair. Belly breathing means:
- Take a long breath. As you inhale, become aware of the forward movement and expansion of your abdomen.
- After inhaling, try to hold your breath for the same amount of time it took you to inhale.

- After holding your breath, exhale. Try to make your exhalation twice as long as your inhalation. As you exhale, become aware of pulling your belly inward, pulling your belly toward your spine.
- Repeat seven times.

Your breathing should be in a 1:1:2 rhythm.

For example, your inhale is 4 seconds, your breath hold is also 4 seconds, and your exhale is 8 seconds. If, in the beginning, it is a challenge for you to establish a uniform breathing rhythm, feel free to breathe in a rhythm that is natural to you. Over time, through practice, you will be able to become aware of the correct way of breathing.

This breathing rhythm is also applied when breathing with the lungs and the tops of the lungs.

Lung breathing – In this way of breathing, focus on what is happening in your lungs. Place your palms on your chest, with the left palm over the left lung and the right palm over the right lung. Lung breathing means:

- When inhaling, focus on the expansion of your lungs to the side.
- When breathing with your lungs, don't breathe with your stomach.
- If you feel the expansion of your stomach, stop inhaling.
- The breath hold should be the same length as the inhalation.
- Exhalation should be twice as long as inhalation.
- Repeat seven times.

Breathing with the tops of the lungs - Breathing with the tops of the lungs means you breathe very shallowly; unfortunately, this is the most common form of breathing for most people. The main reasons for this way of breathing are:

- Constant exposure to stress
- Unhealthy way of consuming food (so-called air swallowing - insufficiently chewing the food you eat)
- Unconscious breathing

Breathing with the tops of the lungs:

- Place your fingers on your shoulders or collarbones.

- Be aware of the lifting of your shoulders or collarbones when you inhale.
- Your inhale and breath hold should be the same length.
- Don't breathe with the lungs, only with the tops of the lungs.
- Make your exhalation twice as long as your inhalation.
- Repeat seven times.

After breathing in segments, you will combine these three breaths into one; this combined breathing is part of the chair yoga practice.

During three-layer breathing, you will become aware of the expansion of the stomach and lungs and the lifting of the tops of the lungs during one breath. Place your hands on your knees when you practice three-layer breathing.

Breathing in segments can be done every time before the start of your chair yoga practice (from 3 to 7 times for each position, depending on the time you have available that day). Practice the complete three-layer breathing during your yoga chair practice.

Breathing to strengthen the body's will and resistance

You can practice this breathing technique before starting your yoga chair practice, as it will strengthen your will, especially on days when you are not completely ready for your practice.

It is when you exercise the least that your body needs the most physical activity. By applying this breathing technique, you will never miss a single day of exercise.

If you want your physical health to be at an enviable level, I recommend practicing this technique daily, as soon as you get up.

The breathing technique:

- Keep your back straight; resting it on the back of a chair or bed if you practice it as soon as you wake up.
- Place your hands in a position that is natural to you. There is no improper positioning of the hands.
- Breathe in through your nose as deeply as you can.

- Holding your breath, lower your chin toward your sternum. Make contact between your chin and sternum if you can. If you can't, it's perfectly fine to point your chin towards your sternum.
- Hold your breath for as long as you feel comfortable.
- Exhaling through your nose, lift your chin. Exhale as much as you can.
- Repeat this breathing technique at least three times. There is no maximum.

Sound S breathing - relaxation of the nervous system

By practicing sound S, you can completely relax your nervous system and strengthen your nerves easily and simply.

You can practice this breathing technique before starting your chair yoga practice to calm your nervous system and draw focus to the practice.

You can also practice this breathing technique in stressful situations (traffic jams, discussions with close people, important business meetings, etc.).

Sound-S breathing:

- Keep your back straight.
- You can slightly tilt your chin toward your sternum. There is no need to touch the sternum.
- Take a deep breath through your nose.
- After inhaling, exhale with a sound S through the mouth, resting the tip of the tongue on the front inside of the upper teeth.
- Exhale the audible S for as long as you can.
- Repeat at least three times.

If you practice this breathing in moments when you are under stress, you can freely practice it more than three times, until you feel calm and relaxed.

Tips for Protecting Your Body and Warming Up

Before starting your practice, it is very important to properly protect your body during exercise. This way, you make it easier to remain consistent in your practice and to successfully achieve your desired weight.

Try to adhere to the following 11 tips to protect your body during exercise:

- **Inform your personal physician about your desire to start a chair yoga practice** – Your physician is most familiar with your health condition, and you need their consent as far as exercise is concerned.

  Familiarize your physician with the exercises you will practice. They will have better knowledge on what exercises you can perform without jeopardizing your health.

- **Wear appropriate clothes and shoes** – Do not wear clothes that are too tight or too loose. Wear clothing you feel comfortable in. The same applies to footwear; never use sneakers that are not your size.

- **Exercise in an appropriate space** - The space you set aside for exercise should not be too small and should have at least one window to ensure uninterrupted air flow. The space in which you practice must be clutter-free.

- **Be completely mindful during the exercise** - This means that you follow the instructions carefully during the execution of each position. Breathe consciously to perform the positions with more focus.

- **Be aware of your body's limitations** - Never try to go beyond your body's comfort level during exercise. If you do this, it is very easy to get injured and end your chair yoga practice.

- **Warm up your body** - By warming up properly, you will prevent possible injuries. Later in the chapter, you will learn about basic warm-up exercises.

- **Hydrate your body** - Always keep a bottle of water with you. By regularly hydrating your body, you will prevent dehydration and possible dizziness. Dizziness can cause a possible fall, so regular hydration is a **must!**

- **Pay attention to the position of your knees** - While sitting on a chair, your knees should be exactly above your ankles. You must not allow your knees to be in front of your ankles.

- **Pay attention to the position of your feet** - Both feet should have firm and secure support on the yoga mat. Become aware of the contact of the toes, soles, and heels with the yoga mat.
- **Pay attention to your back** - Your back should be completely straight during the exercise and supported by the back of the chair unless otherwise stated in the exercise instructions.
- **No rocking in the chair** - You must not rock in the chair while practicing the position. Perform each position slowly and with great focus.

Warm up your body properly

Before any physical activity, you should properly warm up your body. A proper warm-up is very important for your joints, skeletal, and nervous systems.

Warm-up movements will not take more than five minutes, so you should never skip warm-up exercises before starting your chair yoga routine.

Do not rush through the warm-up exercises; perform them with focus.

If you do not do the warm-up exercises in the manner and with the dynamics described, you risk getting injured due to insufficient warm-up.

The warm-up exercises described below are very easy and simple to perform. Accordingly, you can do all the warm-up exercises before every practice.

Of course, if you can perform more repetitions for a certain exercise, feel free to do so.

Remember, the warm-up will not take more than five minutes, so don't skip it!

Cat cow pose

Thanks to this simple movement, you will feel relief in your back, especially in the lumbar area.

Sit on a chair with your feet firmly positioned on the yoga mat hip-width apart and your palms on your knees (your arms are outstretched).

Start this movement with a complete three-layer inhalation while sitting upright.

As you exhale, drop your chin toward your sternum, lowering your head and creating a curve in your upper back.

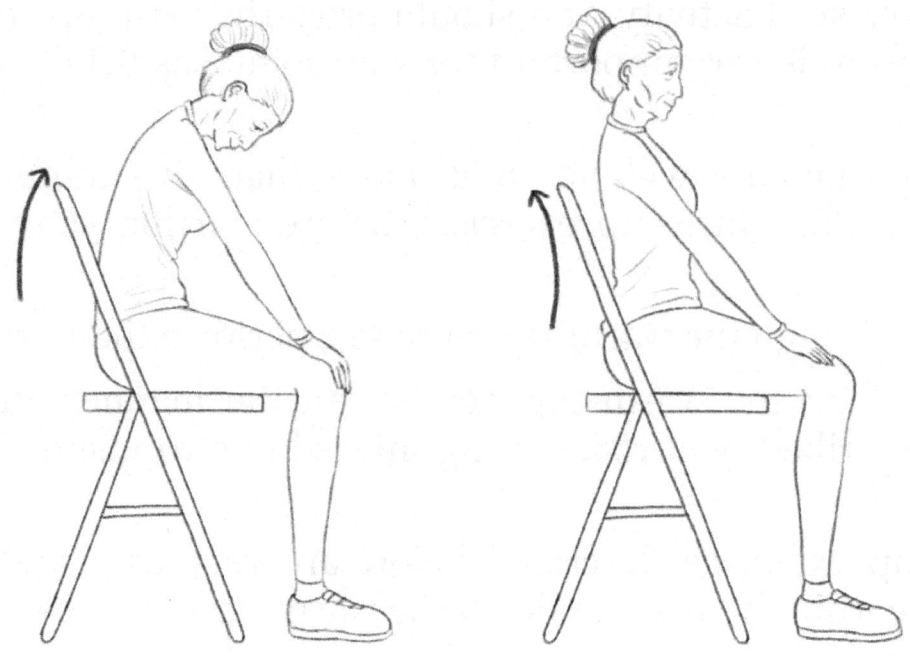

With an inhale, lift your head and chin back to the starting position, and your chest expands forward. Your back will gently stretch as you inhale.

Repeat five times!

****

FREE GIFT #2: EXCLUSIVE ACCESS TO VIDEO TUTORIALS

For detailed video demonstrations of every exercise featured in this book (and other free bonuses), visit **bit.ly/YogaBonuses**

These video guides are carefully created to help you perform each movement accurately and safely, enhancing your ability to follow along and benefit from these exercises.

You can also scan the QR code with your phone camera if you prefer not to type. It's absolutely free.

I hope you find it helpful and enjoyable.

****

Wrist rotation

While sitting with your back straight in a chair, raise your arms at chest height and interlace your fingers.

Do between five and ten circles first to the right, then repeat to the left.

While performing these movements, breathe in three layers.

Thanks to these movements, you will establish better circulation in your fingers, palms, and hands, and you will achieve the necessary mobility and flexibility in your wrists.

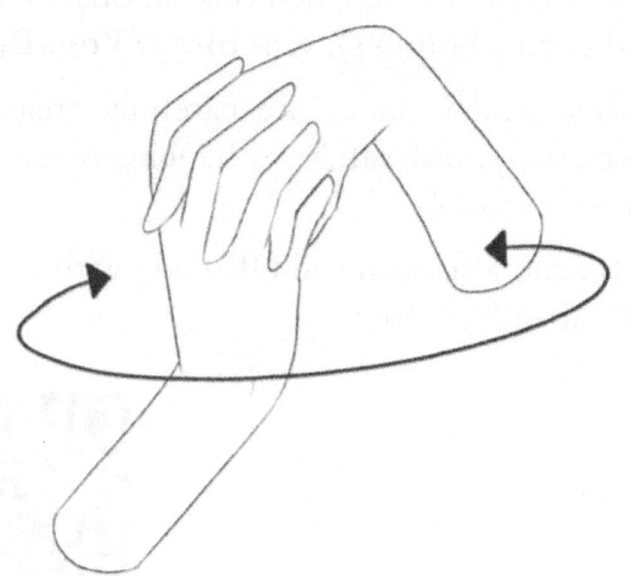

Toe rotations

While sitting with your back straight in a chair, lift the heel of your right foot off the yoga mat and do five to ten circles, first inward, then outward.

After completing the circles, place your right foot on the yoga mat and lift your left foot. Perform the same number of circles.

During these movements, breathe in three layers.

This movement will improve circulation in the toes, soles, heels, and ankles, and will improve your flexibility and mobility.

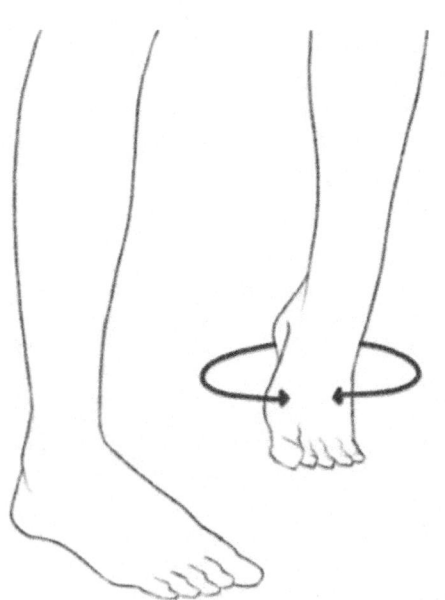

Shoulder circles

While sitting with your back straight, perform five to ten circles with your shoulders, first forward, then backward.

During this movement, breathe in three layers.

Thanks to these movements, you will warm up your entire shoulder girdle, shoulder blades, and the space between them.

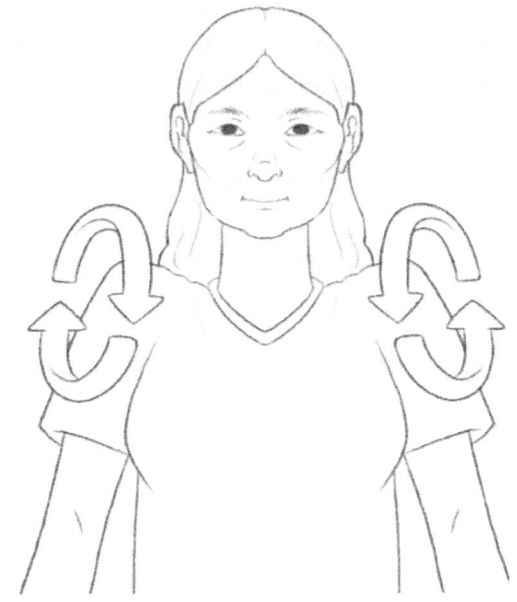

Pelvic tilt

Thanks to this movement, you will be more aware of the movement of your pelvis and thus perform all the positions in your practice with greater ease.

It will also avoid injuries that can occur due to insufficient movement in the pelvic area.

While performing this movement, sit on the chair with your back straight and your feet firmly planted on the yoga mat hip width apart.

To become more aware of the movement, place your palms on your stomach.

As you inhale, your pelvis will move forward, while as you exhale, it will move backwards.

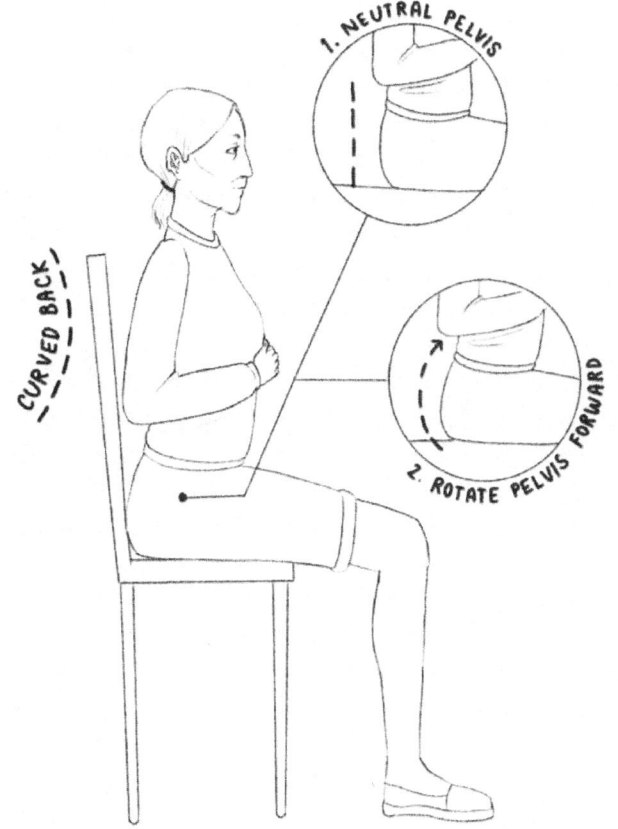

With your palms placed on your stomach, you will remain aware of your breathing and the movement of your pelvis.

During this movement, breathe with your stomach. That's why I recommend placing your palms on your stomach to ensure proper breathing. Perform ten forward and backward pelvic movements.

Neck stretches

When performing neck movements, sit in the chair with your back completely straight and breathe from the stomach.

The first movement involves turning your head to the right and pointing your chin towards your right shoulder. Stay in this position for five inhalations and exhalations.

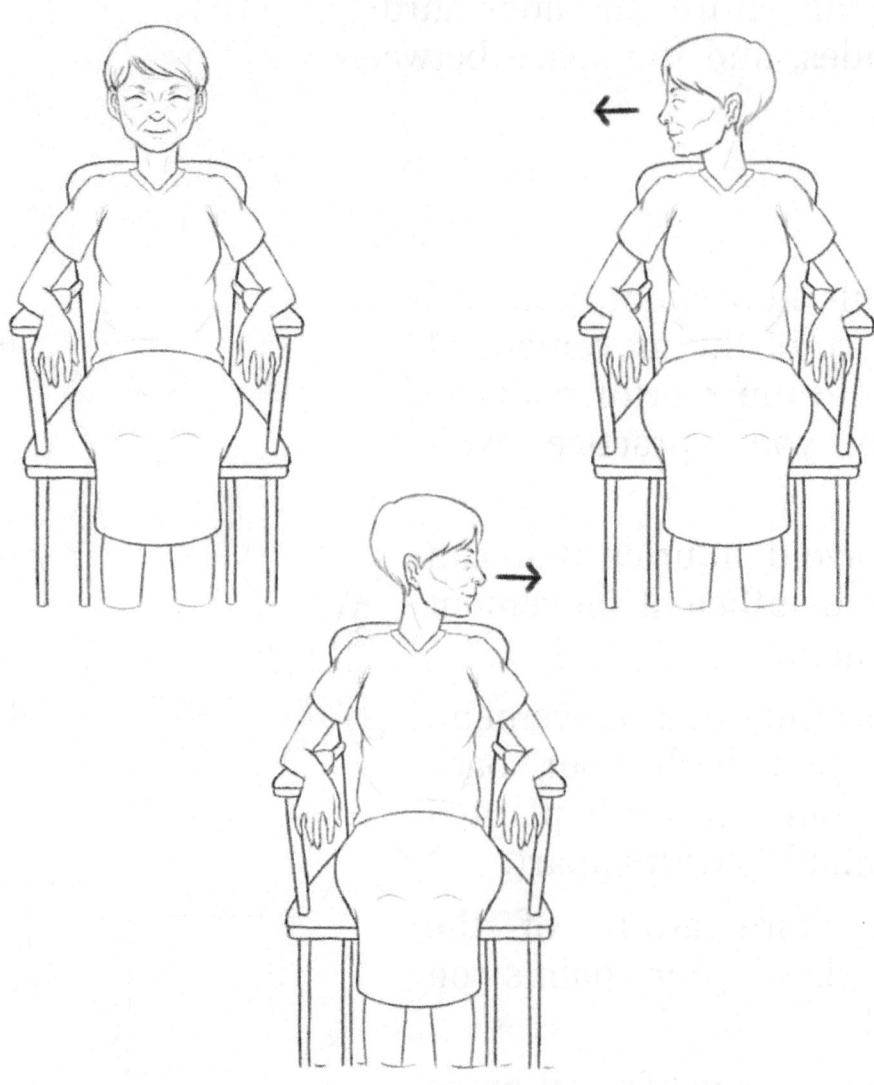

Repeat on the left side.

The second movement involves extending your left arm downward as your right ear aligns with your right shoulder. Stay in this position for five inhalations and exhalations.

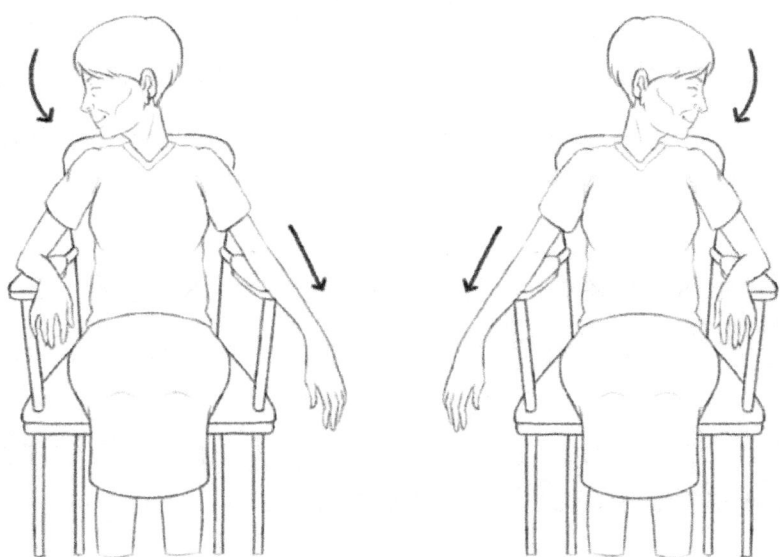

Repeat on the other side.

Thanks to these movements, the blood circulation in your neck will improve. You will stretch your neck, the neck vertebrae and neck veins, and warm up the neck muscles.

In this chapter, you learned how to:
- Reorganize and change your way of thinking with the goal of filling your chair yoga practice with mindfulness.
- Choose appropriate equipment and space for your practice.
- Apply basic breathing techniques.
- Apply 11 tips to make your practice safer.
- Practice easy and simple warmup movements.

In the next chapter, we will explore postures that aim at improving flexibility, mobility, core balance, digestion, and metabolism.

You will find out how these positions contribute to weight loss if you practice them regularly.

Let's step into the practice together!

CHAPTER 3:
18 Simple but Effective Chair Yoga Poses

"Efficiency is doing things right. Effectiveness is doing the right things."
- Peter Drucker

Because chair yoga features low impact exercises, it is the perfect choice for your joints and for establishing the necessary mobility and flexibility in your body.

Through a regular chair yoga practice, your body will burn more calories than usual, which is essential for weight loss.

Thanks to chair yoga, you will increase muscle tone, which can lead to an increase in metabolic rate over time, facilitating weight loss.

In this chapter, you will be introduced to effective chair yoga poses that will improve your mobility and flexibility, strengthen your core, balance, and establish better functioning of your metabolism and digestive system.

Poses for mobility and flexibility

When your body has the necessary mobility and flexibility, you will:

- Reduce the risk of injuries.
- Greatly reduce or eliminate existing pain.
- Improve your posture and body alignment.
- Increase your range of motion, reducing the possibility of falling.
- Establish better circulation throughout the body.
- Recover faster from slight injuries.
- Improve your quality of life.
- Age gracefully.

The poses found in this chapter can be combined in any way you want.

For example, you can do two poses for mobility and flexibility, three poses for the core, one for metabolism, and two for balance.

You get to choose which poses to perform each day. Over time, you will become aware of the poses that suit your body on any day.

In the beginning, I advise you to stay in the poses for lower breath cycles with the aim of going through all the poses. This will help you understand the benefits of each pose.

Seated Mountain Pose

This pose will provide you with:

- Better stability and grounding
- Greater hip flexibility
- Better posture
- Better breathing
- Calmness of mind and greater presence

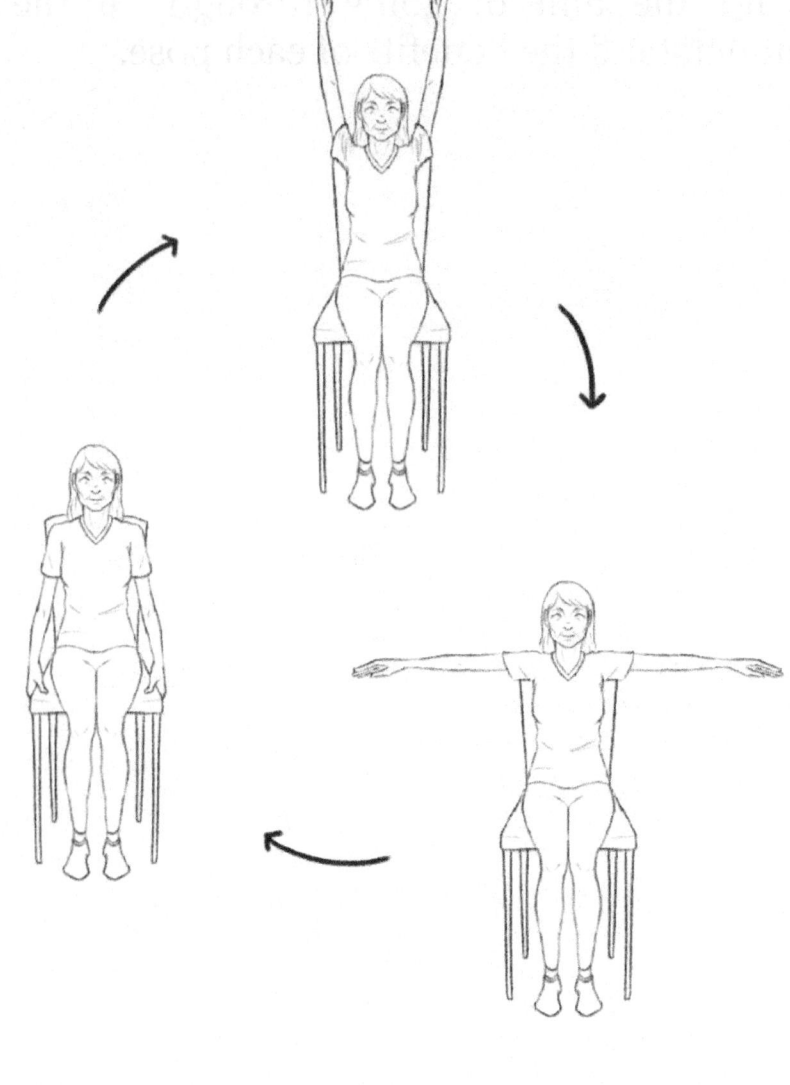

Instructions, step-by-step:

- Sit in a chair with your back straight, leaning against the back of the chair.
- Place your feet firmly on the yoga mat. Your feet can be together or hip-width apart (choose the position you feel more stable in).
- With a triple inhale (three-layer as explained in Chapter 2) raise your arms above your head, stretching them as far as you can. Stay in this position for 3 to 5 breaths. Stretch your spine upwards throughout the exercise; this will improve your posture and the flexibility of your spine.
- With the next breath, lower your arms to the sides at shoulder height, stretching your arms to the sides. This way, you open your shoulders and shoulder blades. Stay in this position for 3 to 5 breaths.
- With an exhalation, lower your arms to the sides of your body.

Seated Forward Bend

This pose will:
- Stretch the hamstrings
- Open the hips
- Improve digestive function
- Improve spine flexibility
- Improve posture
- Improve blood circulation
- Have a therapeutic effect on sciatica (if you are dealing with sciatica)
- Relax the nervous system

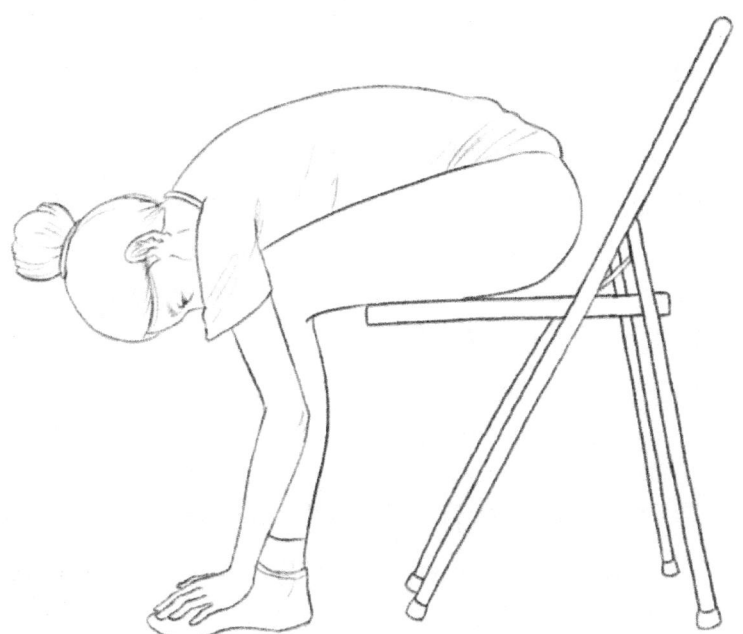

Instructions, step-by-step:
- Sit on the front of the chair with your back straight. Your feet are firmly planted hip-width apart on the yoga mat.
- Inhale, and with an exhale without moving your hips, begin to lower your upper body towards your thighs.
- If your body allows, bring your upper body into contact with your thighs. If you are unable to make contact, stop your upper body in a position that is comfortable for you.
- With your hands, embrace your feet, ankles, or calves, all to gently stretch your back and groin.
- Stay in that position, breathing in three layers, for 3 to 5 breaths.
- After that, take a breath and slowly return to the starting position.

Seated Butterfly Stretch

This pose will help:
- Stretch your groin
- Improve blood circulation
- Open the hips
- Improve digestive functioning
- Improve posture
- Establish nervous balance

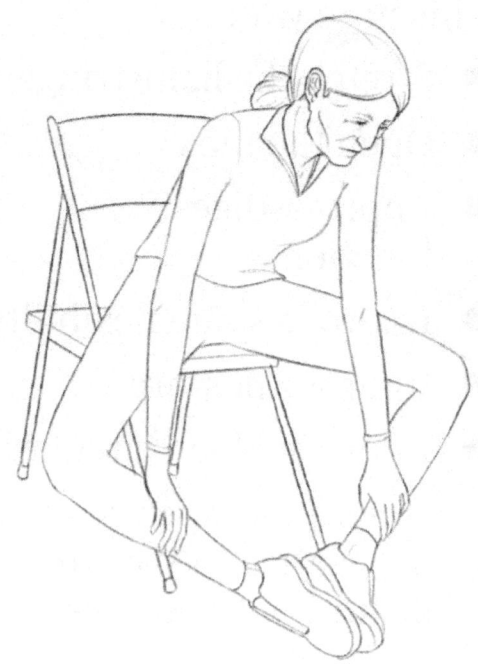

Instructions, step-by-step:
- Sit on the front of the chair with your back straight.
- Bring your heels together; if you can, connect your feet and toes.
- Move your knees as far as you can to the side.
- When you can no longer bring your knees down to the side, lower your upper body and grasp your feet, ankles, or calves with your hands.
- From that position, if your body allows, move your knees down to the side a little more. This gently opens your hips and inner thighs.
- Stay in the position for 3 to 5 breaths.
- Inhale and return to the starting position.

Seated Pigeon Pose

This pose will help:
- Improve hip flexibility
- Relax the lower back
- Stimulate the digestive system
- Improve posture
- Improve blood circulation
- Ease tension in the sciatic nerve

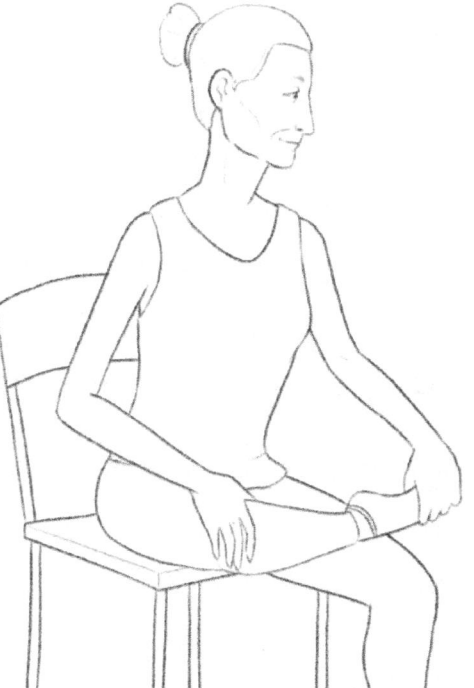

Instructions, step-by-step:
- Sit on the front of the chair seat with your back straight. Both your feet are firmly on the yoga mat, about hip-width apart.
- Lift your right foot and place it on your left knee. If you can't lift your right foot high enough to place on your left knee, lift it as far as your body allows, holding your right foot with your left palm.
- In both variations, place your right palm on your right knee.
- Gently push your right knee down with your right palm, but ensure you remain comfortable. This move stretches your right hip and gluteus.
- Stay in the final position for 3 to 5 breaths.
- Inhale and return to the starting position by placing your right foot on the yoga mat.
- Repeat on the left side.

Poses to strengthen the core

A strong core is very important if you want to lose weight. The main indicators that point to the connection between a strong core and weight loss are:

- **Increased overall strength and endurance** - As you become stronger, you will be able to burn calories more easily during exercise.

- **Better posture and alignment** - Thanks to a better body posture, you will be able to activate your body much more easily and simply during physical activities, and at the same time, you will reduce the risk of possible injuries.

- **Increased calorie consumption** - As you build a strong core, you will also burn calories faster. Accordingly, core-strengthening postures in your chair yoga practice will be an integral part of your daily practice.

- **Better breathing and circulation** - As you develop a strong core, your belly breathing will improve. Better belly breathing means better circulation; better circulation means more endurance, which certainly results in faster calorie burning.

- **Decreased lower back pain** - A strong core will allow you to reduce or eliminate lower back pain. When you no longer have lower back pain, the intensity of your physical activity will improve, which is extremely important if you want to lose weight.

Seated Side Stretch

This pose will help:
- Improve back flexibility
- Relax the lower back
- Fine stretch the intercostal muscles
- Ease tension in the shoulders
- Increase detoxification by stimulating the digestive organs
- Improve kidney function
- Increase lung capacity
- Increase energy in the whole body

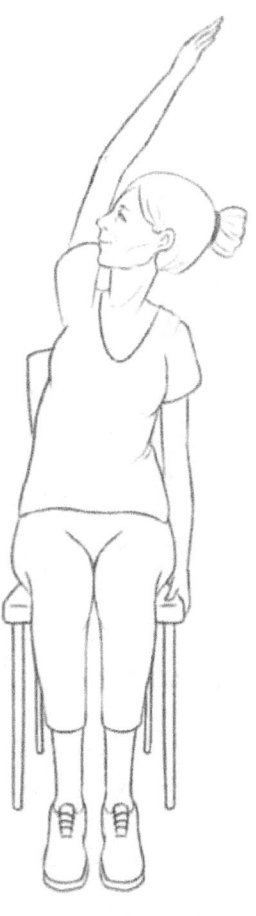

Instructions, step-by-step:
- Sit on a chair with your back straight. You can lean against the back of the chair if it's more comfortable.
- Firmly plant your feet on the yoga mat, keeping your feet and knees together.
- With an inhale, raise your right arm above your body and stretch it as high as you can towards the ceiling.
- For more stability while performing this position, you can grab the seat of the chair with your left hand.
- Stay in this position for 3 to 5 breaths.
- Be aware of the stretch along the right waist and the fine extension of the right hip.
- Activate your core during the pose.
- Repeat the same movement on the left side.

Seated Leg Lifts

This pose will help:
- Stretch the hip flexor
- Strengthen core
- Strengthen legs
- Improve functioning of the digestive organs
- Improve blood circulation, especially in the lower extremities
- Improve posture

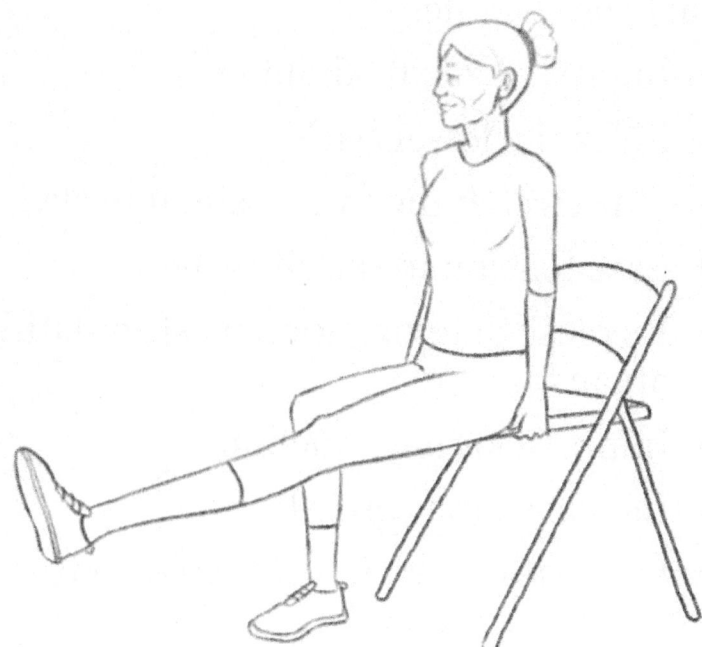

Instructions, step-by-step:
- Sit with your back straight at the center of the chair with your feet firmly planted on the yoga mat.
- Hold on to the sides of the chair with both hands.
- Inhale in the position, and with an exhale, lift the right leg up. If you can, raise your leg high so that your hip, knee, and ankle align. Activate your core. With an exhalation, lower the leg.
- Repeat on the left side.
- Alternately, perform 5 to 10 repetitions.

If you think you're up for a bigger challenge, try a static variation of this exercise. When you raise your leg, try to keep it in position for 3 to 5 breaths.

If you manage to do this variation, try lifting both legs at the same time.

Seated Boat Pose

This pose will help:
- Strengthen core
- Strengthen hip flexors
- Strengthen the back
- Improve balance and flexibility of the whole body
- Strengthen quadriceps and thighs
- Improve functioning of the digestive organs
- Calm of the nervous system
- Improve concentration and focus

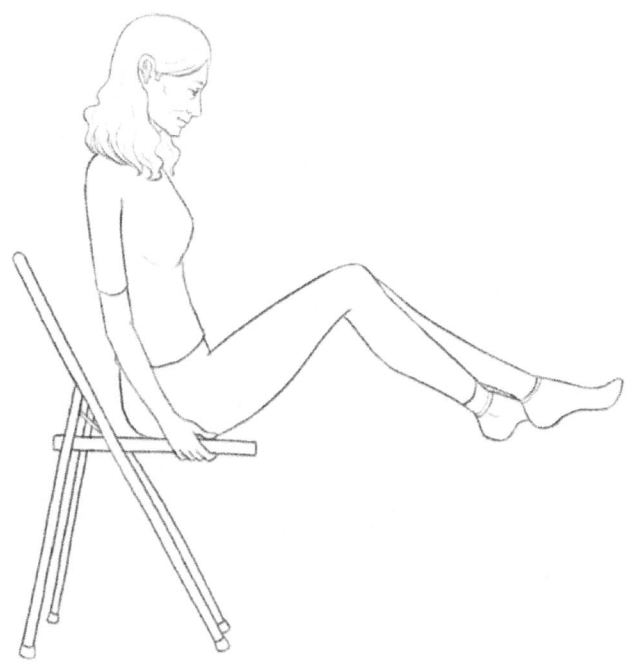

Instructions, step-by-step:
- Sit at the center of the chair with your feet firmly planted on the yoga mat.
- Grab both sides of the chair firmly with your hands.
- Lean back slowly, all within the limits of your body. It is important to remain stable in your position. If you feel that you are losing support and stability, it is a sign that you have leaned back too far.
- Inhale in the position, and exhaling, gently lift your legs off the yoga mat as far as you can. Engage your core as you lift your legs.
- Stay in the position for 3 to 5 breaths.

Do not force lifting your legs and staying in the position for a long time; follow the limits of your body's endurance. Only in this way will you avoid injuries, and you will be able to constantly progress in your chair yoga practice.

Seated Bicycle Crunches

This pose will help:
- Strengthen hip flexors
- Define the oblique muscles
- Strengthen core
- Improve back flexibility
- Stimulate faster burning of calories
- Improve coordination and balance

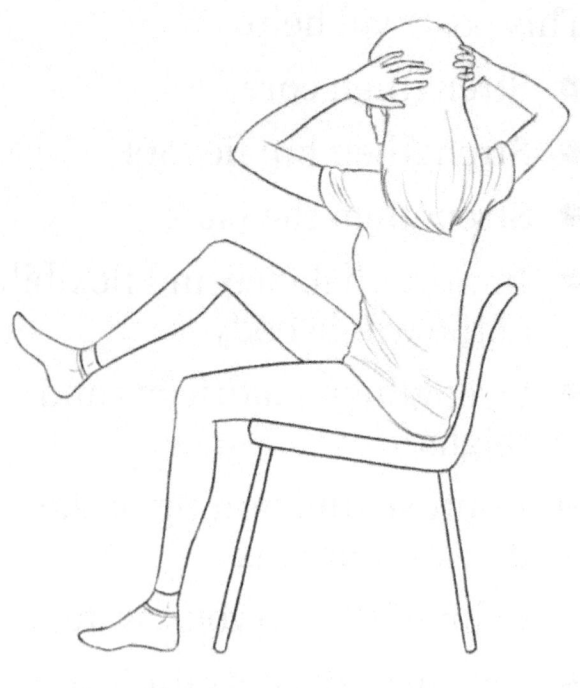

Instructions, step-by-step:
- Sit at the center of the chair with your feet planted hip-width apart on the yoga mat.
- Interlace your fingers and place your palms behind your head.
- Inhale, and with an exhale, lift the right knee and try to make contact between the left elbow and the right knee while rotating your upper body to the right.
- Do it on the left side.
- Alternately, perform 5 to 10 repetitions.

In case you do not have stability in the chair when your hands are behind your head, you can firmly grasp both sides of the chair with your hands. In this variant, you will have the stability you need. When raising your knees, you will only rotate your upper body to the right and left.

Poses for better balance

Thanks to your body's improved balance, you will achieve your desired weight with greater ease.

Improved balance:
- Reduces the risk of injuries.
- Provides better posture, engaging your core more.
- Allows you to have better movement, burning more calories.
- Can speed up your metabolism.

Seated Tree Pose

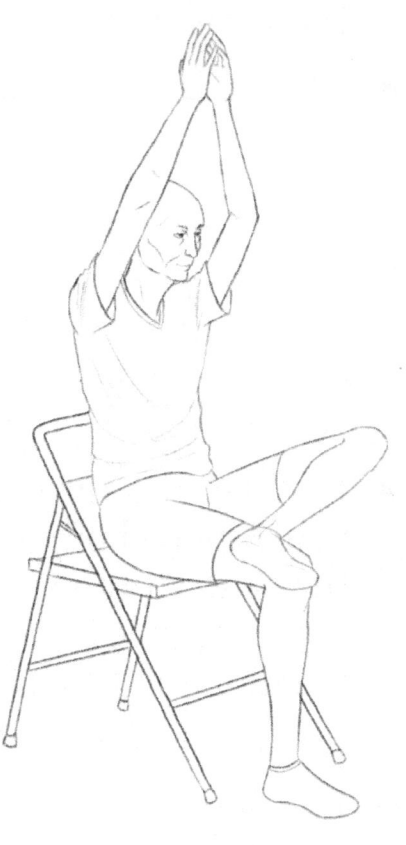

This pose will help:
- Stretch the inner thighs
- Open the hips
- Improve stability and grounding
- Improve posture
- Improve balance
- Improve concentration and focus

Instructions, step-by-step:
- Sit on a chair with your back straight. Your feet are firmly planted on the yoga mat about hip-width apart. If you want, you can rest your back on the back of the chair.
- Lift your right foot and place it on your left knee. If you find it challenging, place your foot on the inside of your left thigh. If you find that challenging, place your right foot on your left ankle.
- Hold on to the sides of the chair with both hands.
- If you feel you have good balance, you can try to do a full pose. Stretch your arms above your head and bring your palms together.
- Stay in the selected position for 3 to 5 breaths.

Seated Chair Twist

This pose will help:
- Improve back mobility
- Stretch hip flexor
- Open the chest
- Improve functioning of the digestive organs
- Improve detoxification
- Strengthen core
- Improve blood circulation
- Relax the nervous system

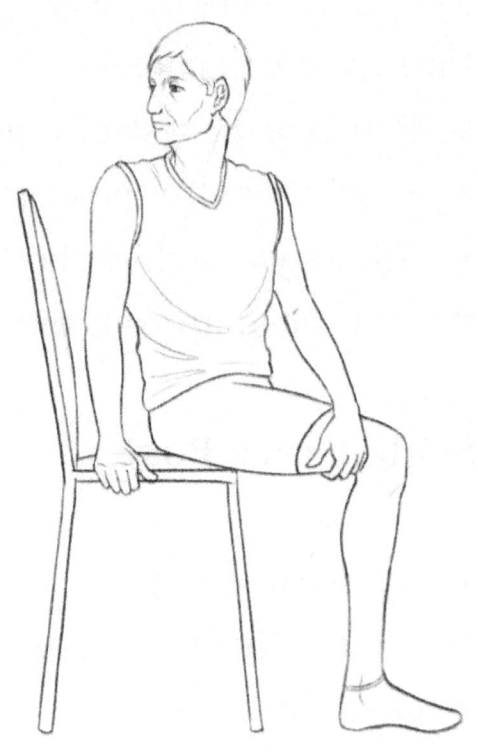

Instructions, step-by-step:
- Sit with your back straight on the front of the chair so that there is space between your glutes and the back of the chair. Plant your feet hip width apart on the yoga mat and place your palms on your knees.
- Perform the three-layer inhalation and with an exhale, gently rotate your upper body to the right, placing the palm of the right hand on the seat, in the space between your glutes and the back of the chair. Place your left palm on the outside of your right knee. Stay in this position for 3 to 5 breaths.
- Inhale and return the upper body and palms to the starting position.
- Repeat the twist on the left side.

Seated Warrior I

This pose will help:
- Strengthen core muscles
- Stretch hip flexor
- Stretch and strengthen arms
- Stretch the waist
- Strengthen legs
- Improve functioning of the digestive organs
- Open the chest
- Improve blood circulation
- Improve balance and body posture

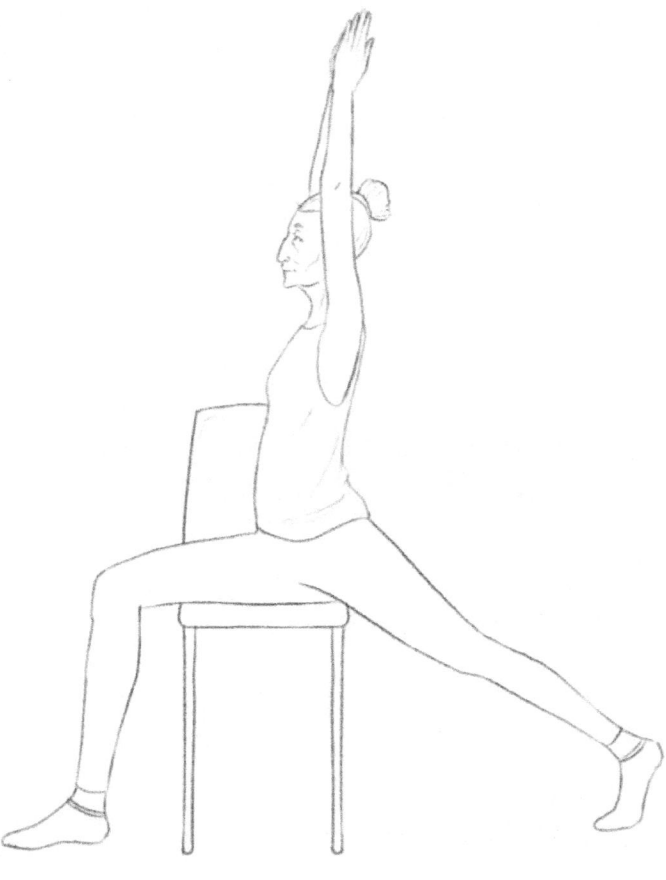

Instructions, step-by-step:
- Sit with your back straight on the chair and your feet hip-width apart on the yoga mat.
- Rotate the left foot ninety degrees to the left. If you can't rotate your foot to ninety degrees, rotate it as far as your body will allow.
- Rotate your upper body to the left.
- Extend the right leg back, point the toes of the right foot and lift the right heel.
- Stretch your arms above your head and bring your palms together.
- Stay in the position for 3 to 5 breaths.
- Repeat the position on the right side.

Chair Side Leg Lifts

This pose will help:
- Strengthen the thighs
- Strengthen the hip abductors
- Strengthen the legs
- Improve hip flexibility
- Stabilize the knee
- Ease standing up and climbing
- Improve circulation, especially in the lower part of the body

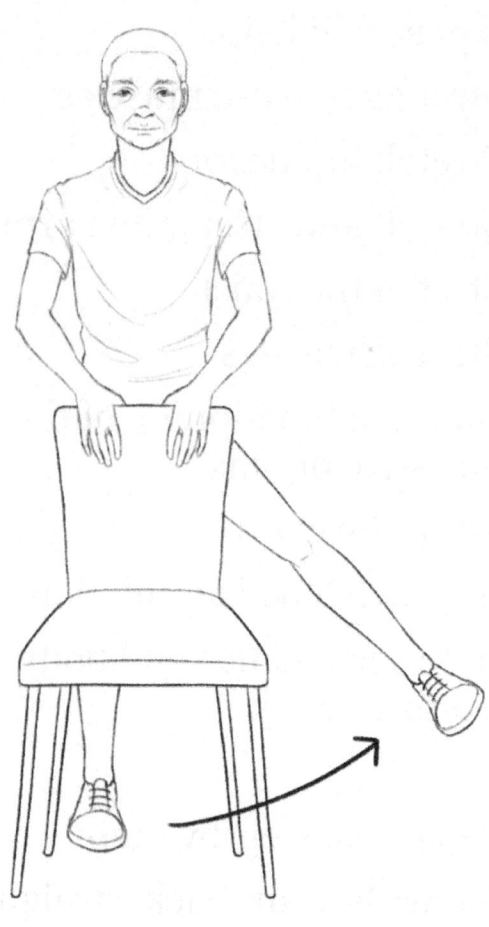

Instructions, step-by-step:
- Stand behind the back of the chair with your back straight and your feet together.
- Hold onto the back of the chair firmly with both hands.
- Inhale, and with an exhale, lift the left leg up to the side as far as you can. Don't force the leg past your body's comfort zone.
- With an inhale, lower the leg to the starting position.
- Repeat on the right side.
- Repeat 5 to 10 times, alternating sides.

Poses to improve metabolism and digestion

Improved metabolism and digestive function are important factors that contribute to achieving your desired weight.

Thanks to proper digestive functioning and improved metabolism, you will:

- Achieve efficient absorption of ingested food.
- Reduce the possibility of accumulating calories.
- Achieve healthy sugar levels.
- Achieve the necessary hormonal balance. This will reduce the need to overeat.
- Have more energy in your body to engage in more vigorous physical activities that will lead to weight loss.

Seated High Knee March

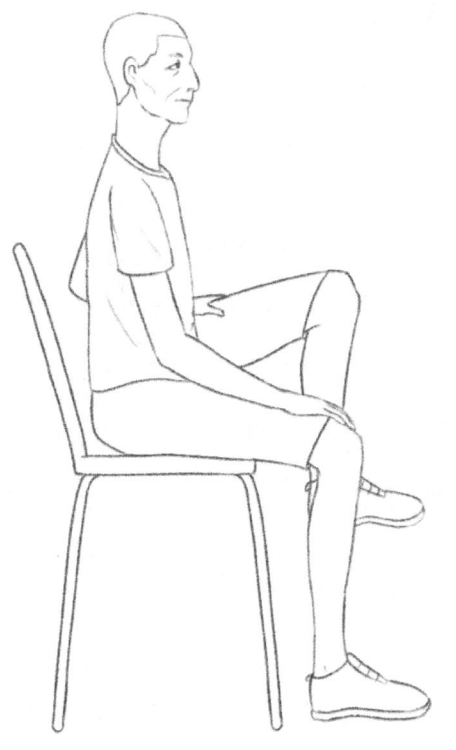

This pose will help:
- Strengthen hip flexors
- Strengthen core
- Strengthen legs
- Stabilize knees
- Improved hip flexibility

Instructions, step-by-step:
- Sit on a chair with your back straight. Your feet are placed hip-width apart on the yoga mat.
- Hold on to the sides of the chair with both hands.
- Inhale, and as you exhale, lift your right leg towards your chest, bending it at the knee. Inhale, then lower the foot to the starting position.
- Do it for the left leg.
- Repeat this movement alternately 5 to 10 times.

Seated Diaphragmatic Breathing

This breathing technique will help:
- Release stress
- Improve breathing (you will increase the capacity of your stomach and lungs)
- Ease coping with anxiety
- Relieve your pain
- Improve functioning of the digestive organs
- Improve sleep quality
- Improve emotional stability
- Improve mental clarity

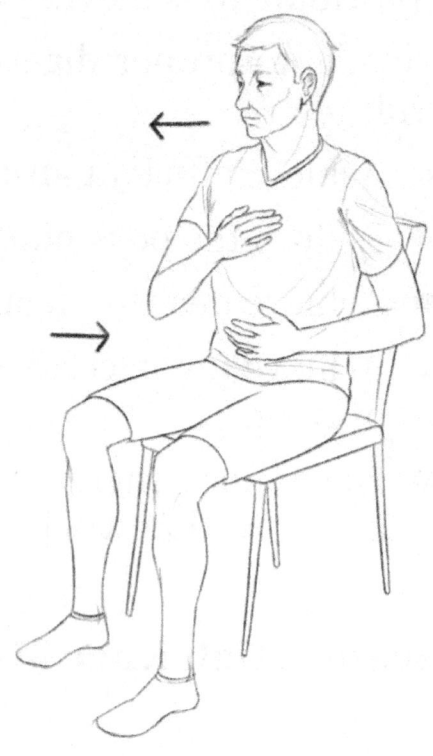

Instructions, step-by-step:
- Sit on a chair with your back straight. Your feet are firmly planted hip-width apart on the yoga mat. If you find it more comfortable, rest your back on the back of the chair.
- Place one palm on your stomach and the other on your chest.
- Take a deep breath and become aware of the expansion of your belly.
- Exhaling, become aware of your belly contracting inward and the movement of the navel towards the spine. Try to make your exhalation twice as long as your inhalation.
- If you like, practice this breathing with your eyes closed to become more aware of diaphragmatic breathing.
- Inhale and exhale through the mouth.
- Practice this breathing technique for about one minute.

Chair High Lunge

This pose will help:
- Stabilize ankle joints
- Strengthen the quadriceps
- Strengthen legs
- Strengthen the core
- Stretch the hip flexor
- Improve balance

Instructions, step-by-step:
- Stand behind a chair with your back straight. Your feet are hip width apart, in line with each other.
- Firmly grab the back of the chair with both hands.
- Inhale, and as you exhale, step your left leg back as far as you can.
- Your right leg is bent at the knee; try to keep your right thigh as level as possible with the yoga mat. Try to keep your left leg fully stretched back (not bent at the knee), and if you can, lift your left heel off the mat.
- If you have no stability, feel free to lower your left heel back onto the yoga mat.
- Respect the limits of your body; do not step back further than your body allows.
- Stay in this position for 3 to 5 breaths.
- Repeat on the opposite side.

This is an easier variation of this position.

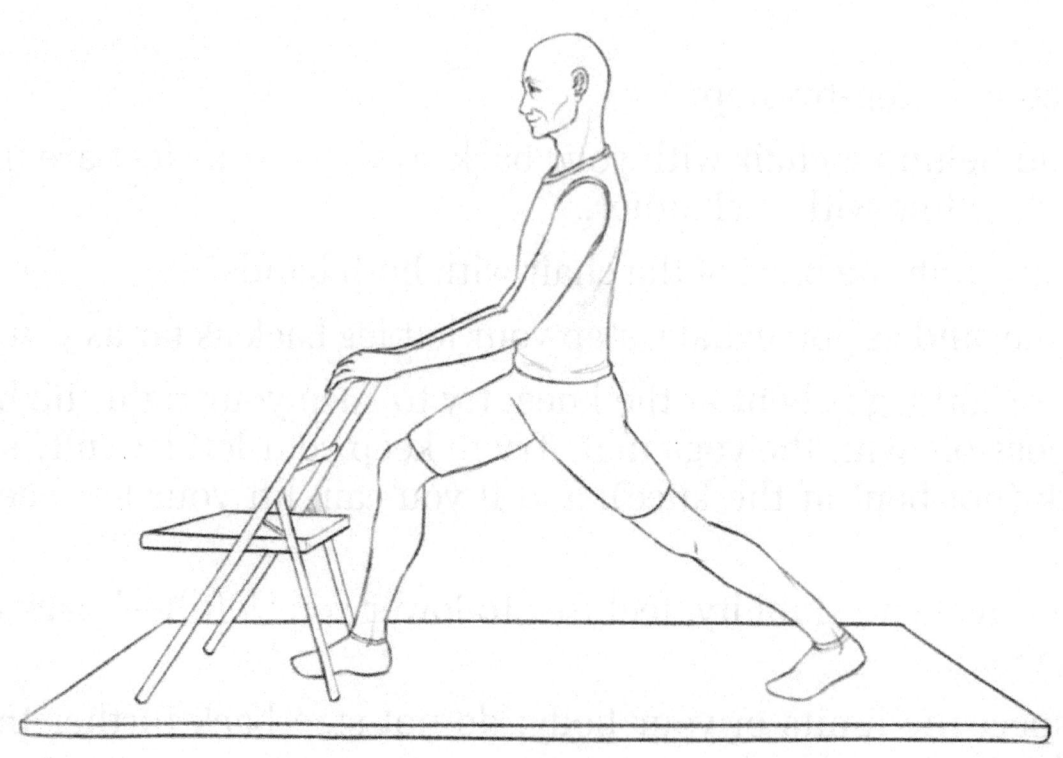

If you have good stability, you can try to perform the full position. When practicing the full pose, it is very important that your chair is stable and firm, placed on the yoga mat and not on the carpet or bare floor.

- Stand in front of a chair with your back straight and your feet hip-width apart.
- Inhale, and as you exhale, lift your left leg and place your left foot on the seat of the chair.
- Your right leg is fully extended, and your right heel is on the yoga mat.
- Place your palms on your left knee.
- Stay in the position for 3 to 5 breaths.
- Repeat on the other side.

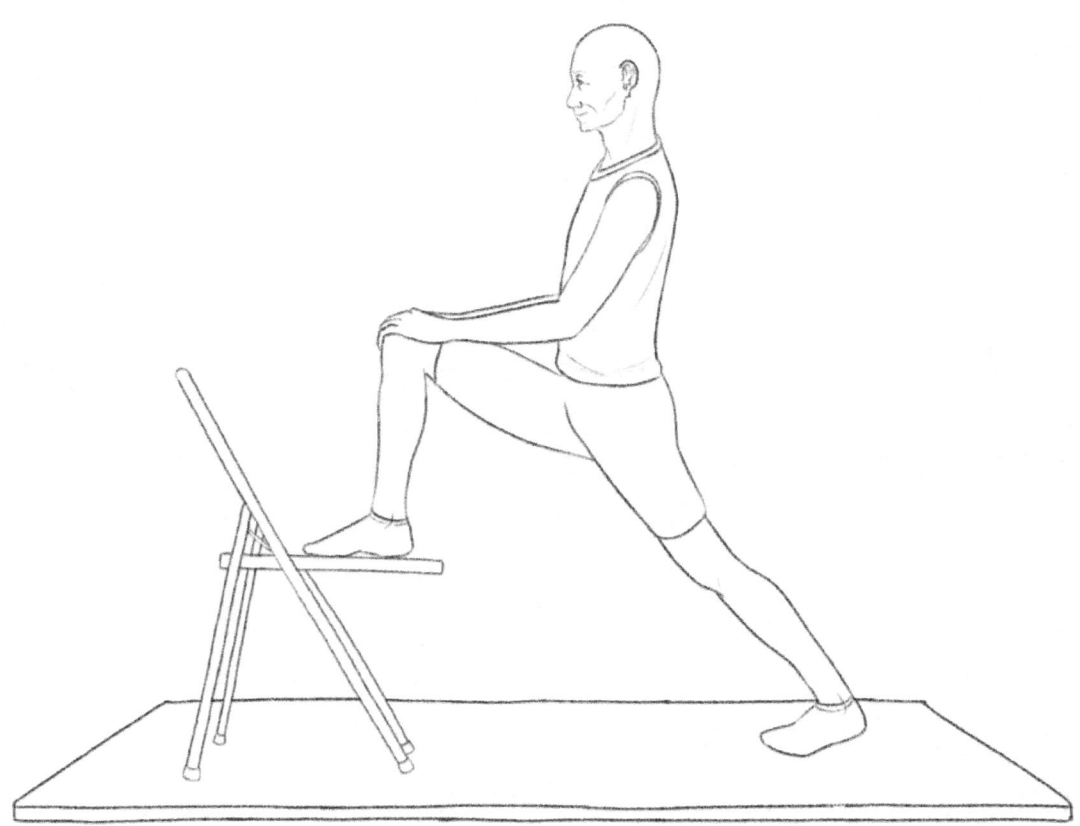

Chair Downward Dog

This pose will help:
- Open the shoulders
- Open the upper back
- Strengthen shoulders and arms
- Relieve discomfort in the back
- Improve core activity
- Stretch the hamstrings
- Open the hips
- Improve blood circulation
- Improve body posture

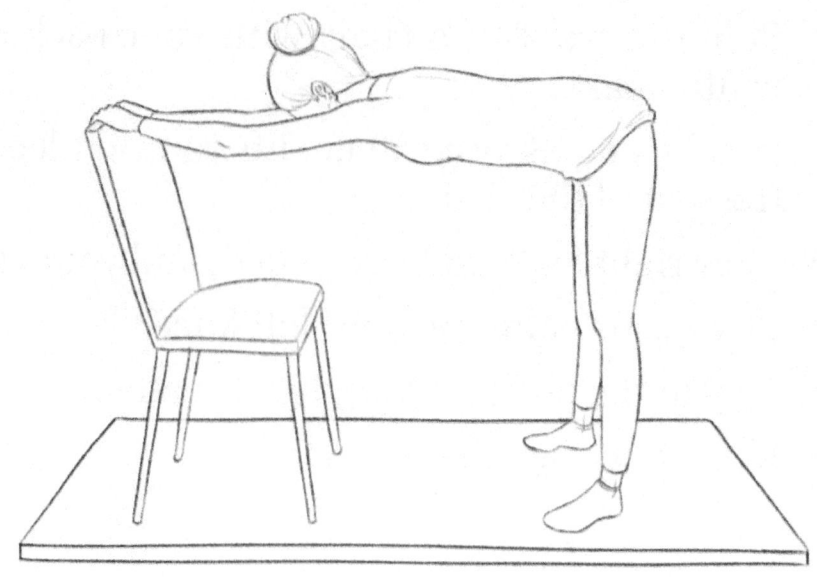

Instructions, step-by-step:
- Stand behind a chair with your feet hip-width apart and your back straight.
  Depending on the proportions of your body, stand far enough behind the chair so that you can fully stretch your arms, firmly grasping the back of the chair.
- Inhale, and with an exhale, slightly bend the upper part of the body, firmly grasping the back of the chair with your hands.
- If necessary, you can slightly bend your knees.
- Try to fully extend your spine and arms.
- Relax your neck; you can gently move your chin towards the sternum.
- Stay in this position for 5 to 10 breaths.

If you want to try a more advanced version, move in front of the chair.
- Facing the chair, stand with your back straight and your feet hip-width apart.
- The proportions of your body will determine how far you stand from the chair.
- Inhale, and with an exhale, slowly bend the upper part of your body until your palms settle on the seat of the chair.
- If necessary, slightly bend your knees.
- Try to keep your spine and arms fully extended.
- You can gently move your chin towards the sternum.
- Stay in this position for 5 to 10 breaths.

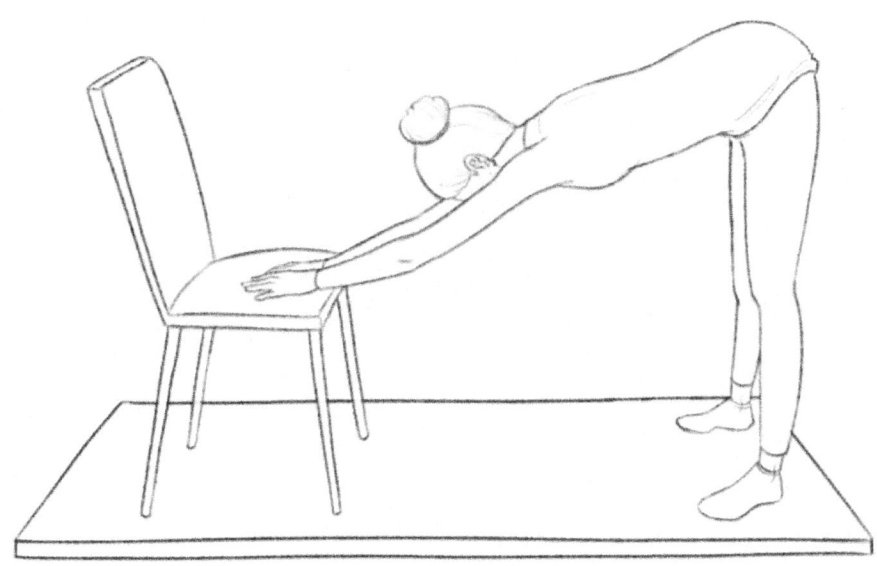

If you are unable to do either variation, you can try a third option - downward dog from a seated position.

- Sit in the center of the chair with your back straight and your feet hip-width apart.
- Stretch your legs, pointing your toes up; your heels will stay on the yoga mat.
- Bend your upper body forward so that your chest is positioned above your thighs.
- Extend your arms up, palms facing forward. Your hands are positioned shoulder-width apart, palms in line with your feet.
- Stay in this position for 5 to 10 breaths.

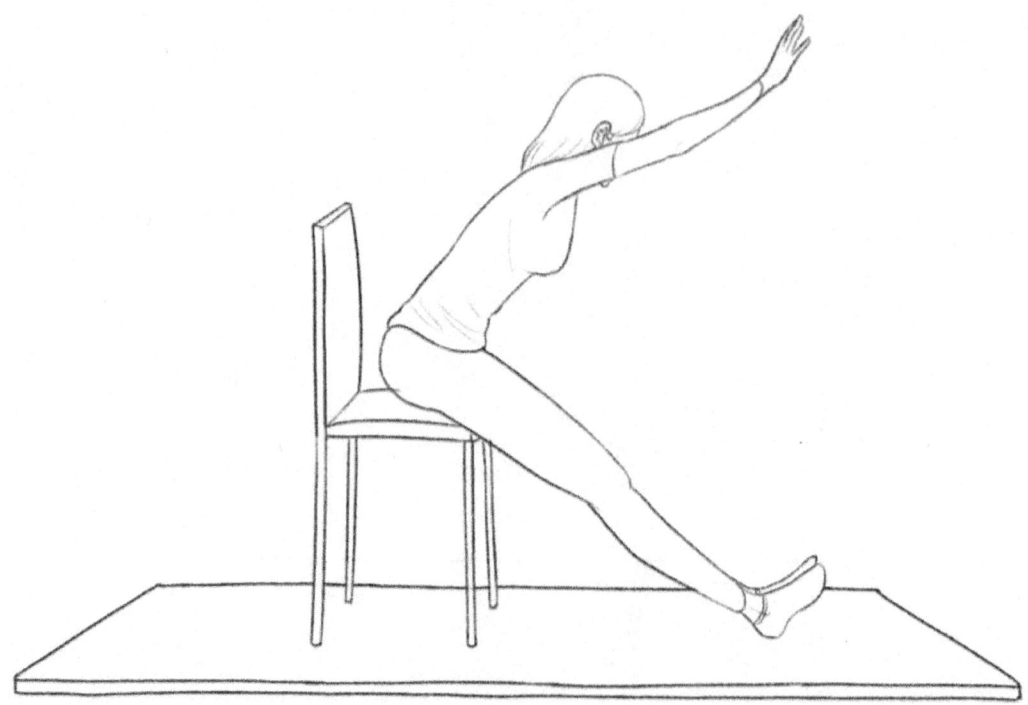

Child's Pose

This pose will help:
- Relax the neck, back, and shoulders
- Stretch the hips
- Ease fatigue recovery
- Establish nervous balance
- Ease relaxation of the whole body
- Improve blood circulation

Instructions, step-by-step:
- Sit at the center of the chair with your back straight and your feet together.
- Inhale, and with an exhale, gently move the upper part of your body downwards.
- If you can, bring your chest into contact with your thighs.
- Hold your legs with your hands wrapped under your knees.
- Relax your neck, rest your chin on your knees if you can, and close your eyes.
- Stay in the position for 5 to 10 breaths.

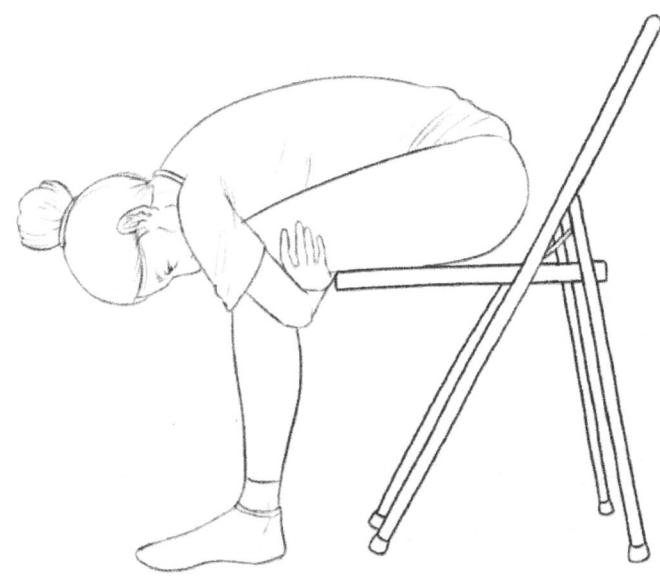

If this variation is challenging, try the next one.
- Sit at the center part of the chair with your back straight and your feet together.
- Inhale, and with an exhale, slowly lower the upper part of your body.
- Rest your elbows on your knees.
- Rest your forehead on your palms.
- Stay in the position for 5 to 10 breaths.

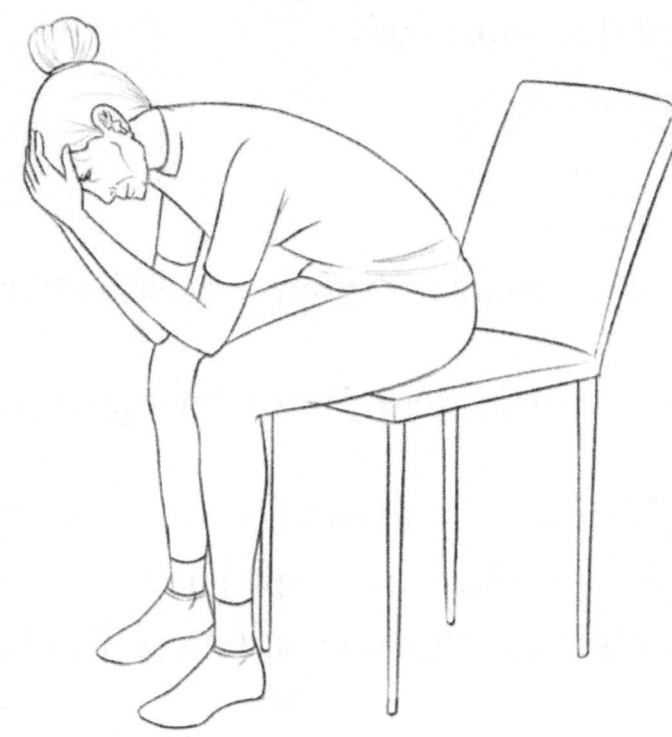

Cobra Pose

This pose will help:
- Improve back flexibility
- Strengthen back muscles
- Improve respiratory function
- Improve functioning of organs in the abdominal cavity
- Improve posture

Instructions, step-by-step:
- Sit at the center of the chair with your back straight and your feet hip-width apart.
- Stretch your arms back, gripping the bottom of the chair's back.
- With an inhale, expand the chest forward and move your head back if you are comfortable. If not, then don't stretch your neck back.
- Exhaling, return to the starting position.
- Repeat this movement 5 to 10 times.

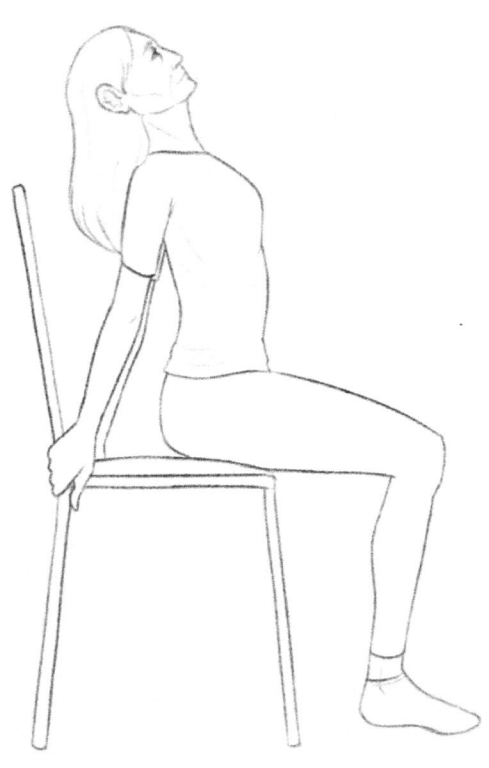

As promised, we have made it through the practice together.

You have learned about, and put into practice, poses that are great for your mobility, flexibility, core, balance, metabolism, and digestion.

The poses practiced in this chapter are very important if you want to achieve weight loss in an easy, simple, and safe way.

The poses outlined in the next chapter are a meaningful progression of the poses found in this chapter.

It is very important to practice the poses found in this chapter regularly. Of course, you get to decide which poses suit you on a particular day.

In the following chapters, I will outline meaningful daily routines to fuel your creativity in designing the sequence of exercises and provide clearly designed pose sequences to promote weight loss.

Make sure that your chair yoga practice goes for at least 10 minutes daily (including warm-up exercises and poses).

If you can spare more than 10 minutes, feel free to extend your chair yoga practice.

MAKE A DIFFERENCE WITH YOUR REVIEW

"Helping one person might not change the whole world, but it could change the world for one person." – **Unknown**

People who give selflessly often find joy in the smallest of gestures. It's in this spirit of kindness and generosity that I ask for a small favor from you.

Would you be willing to extend a helping hand to someone you've never met, with no expectation of recognition?

Who is this person, you wonder? They're a lot like you, or perhaps how you once were. They're eager to learn, improve their health, and regain the flexibility of their youth, but they're unsure where to start.

My mission is to make exercises for seniors something everyone can enjoy and benefit from. To achieve this, I need to reach as many people as possible.

That's where you come in. Most people rely on reviews when choosing a book, so here's my request on behalf of a senior citizen you've never met:

Please take a moment to leave a review for this book.

Your review, which takes less than 60 seconds to write, won't cost you a thing, but it could profoundly impact another senior's life. Your words could help...

...one more grandparent play with their grandkids without pain.

...one more retiree enjoy their golden years to the fullest.

...one more neighbor participate in community activities.

...one more friend share smiles and stories without discomfort.

...one more dream of a healthy, active life come true.

To spread this joy and make a real difference, simply leave your review on Amazon by going to this link: **amzn.to/42eZEud**

Or scan QR code with your camera:

If the thought of helping a fellow senior citizen brings a smile to your face, you're exactly the kind of person I cherish.

Thank you from the bottom of my heart. Let's get back to our journey towards better health and happiness.

Your biggest fan, Michael Smith

PS - Remember, sharing knowledge is one of the best ways to show you care. If you believe this book can help another senior, don't hesitate to pass it along. Your recommendation could be the start of their journey to a healthier, happier life.

CHAPTER 4:
28-Day Challenge to Keep You Motivated

"Believe you can and you are halfway there."

— **Theodore Roosevelt**

The steps and advice in this chapter are aimed at helping you achieve your daily goals, in your chair yoga practice and daily life.

Based on my experience as a personal trainer, I can certainly say that if you want to achieve the goals you for a certain physical activity, you must:

- Start slow
- Follow the advice that will keep you apprised of your progress

By following the steps and following the advice in this chapter, you will stay motivated in the first four weeks of your chair yoga practice.

Why is it important to stay motivated in the first four weeks?

Whenever you start a new activity, the first four weeks represent the **trial period**.

In that time, it is important that your brain, consciousness, and body accept the new activity as something that is useful for your overall development.

Every beginning is difficult, and that's why people falter when starting new things. This means that motivation is a crucial part of the process.

The right motivation will give you the necessary support and encouragement in your journey to achieve your ideal weight.

I am confident that the small steps and tips provided in this chapter will allow you to persevere for the first four weeks of your chair yoga practice. And you can still use the same steps and tips beyond the four weeks.

After the fourth week, everything will be much easier. Activities that may have seemed challenging at first will become an integral part of your daily activities.

Your lifestyle will experience a positive change!

The following detailed plan will accompany you for the first four weeks of your chair yoga practice.

Every week, the plan will be built up to ensure constant progress. The goal of this is to keep you motivated in the first four weeks of chair yoga practice.

FIRST WEEK

Throughout the first week, your chair yoga practice should only include poses for mobility and flexibility from Chapter 3:

1. Seated Mountain Pose
2. Seated Forward Bend
3. Seated Butterfly Stretch
4. Seated Pigeon Pose

Every day during the first week, do all the mobility and flexibility poses.

Try to increase the number of repetitions (for dynamic poses) or number of breaths (for static poses) for each pose by one more from the second to the seventh day.

If an exercise (like seated mountain pose) requires moving your joints through ranges of motion by using combined movements performed at controlled speeds – this is dynamic stretching.

If an exercise (like seated forward bend) requires stretching a muscle to the point where you feel mild discomfort and holding that stretch without moving – this is static stretching.

For example, if on the 1st day you stayed in a certain pose for 1 inhalation and exhalations, on the 7th day you should remain in that pose for 7 inhalations and exhalations:

- ☐ DAY 1: 1 repetition
- ☐ DAY 2: 2 repetitions
- ☐ DAY 3: 3 repetitions
- ☐ DAY 4: 4 repetitions
- ☐ DAY 5: 5 repetitions
- ☐ DAY 6: 6 repetitions
- ☐ DAY 7: 7 repetitions

Of course, if you find it challenging or too easy, feel free to change the number of repetitions to honor the limits of your capabilities, depending on your fitness level.

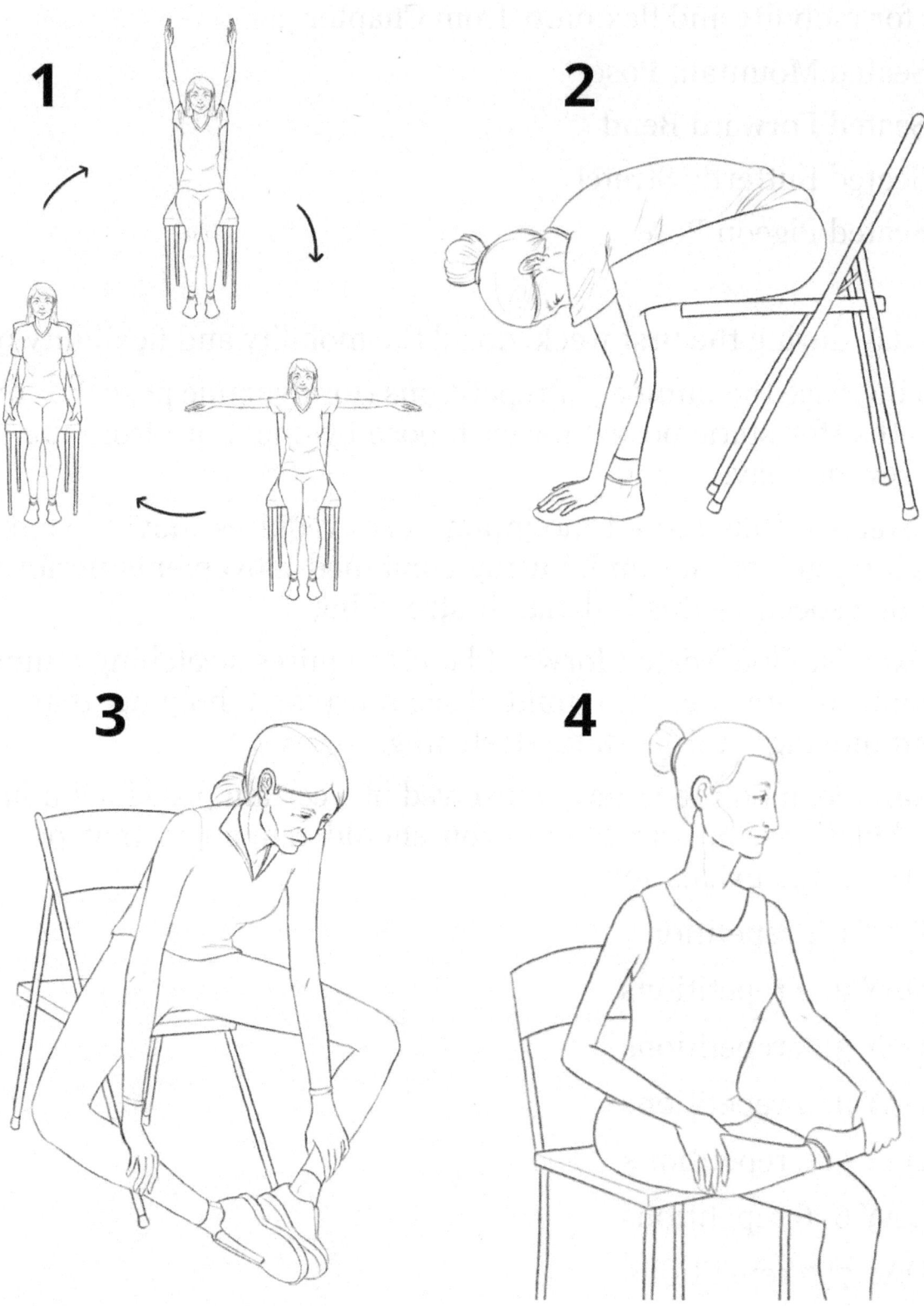

Tips:

- You can have a meal no later than an hour and a half before chair yoga practice (if you don't practice as soon as you get up).
- Try to do your chair yoga practice at the same time every day, without shifting your schedule.
- Stay aware of your breathing. Remember to master the breathing style before the postures.
- If you need to take a day off from exercise and rest, take a Sunday (or another day) off.
- Journal your chair yoga practice. Note how long you exercise each day, what you do, what was easy, and what was challenging.

****

FREE GIFT #3: 28-DAY YOGA CHALLENGE JOURNAL

Kickstart your chair yoga journey with our Printable 28-Day Yoga Challenge Journal. This structured plan will be your companion, helping you track your progress, reflect on your experiences, and stay motivated throughout your journey.

To get your journal, visit **bit.ly/YogaBonuses** and download it (along with other free bonuses).

You can also scan the QR code with your phone camera if you prefer not to type. It's absolutely free.

I hope this journal keeps you inspired and committed to your health and wellness goals.

****

SECOND WEEK

Your yoga practice during the seven days of the second week will include all poses to strengthen your core from Chapter 3:

1. Seated Side Stretch
2. Seated Leg Lifts
3. Seated Boat Pose
4. Seated Bicycle Crunches

Also, from the 8th to the 14th day, try to increase the number of repetitions for core strengthening poses by one more:

- ☐ DAY 8: 1 repetition
- ☐ DAY 9: 2 repetitions
- ☐ DAY 10: 3 repetitions
- ☐ DAY 11: 4 repetitions
- ☐ DAY 12: 5 repetitions
- ☐ DAY 13: 6 repetitions
- ☐ DAY 14: 7 repetitions

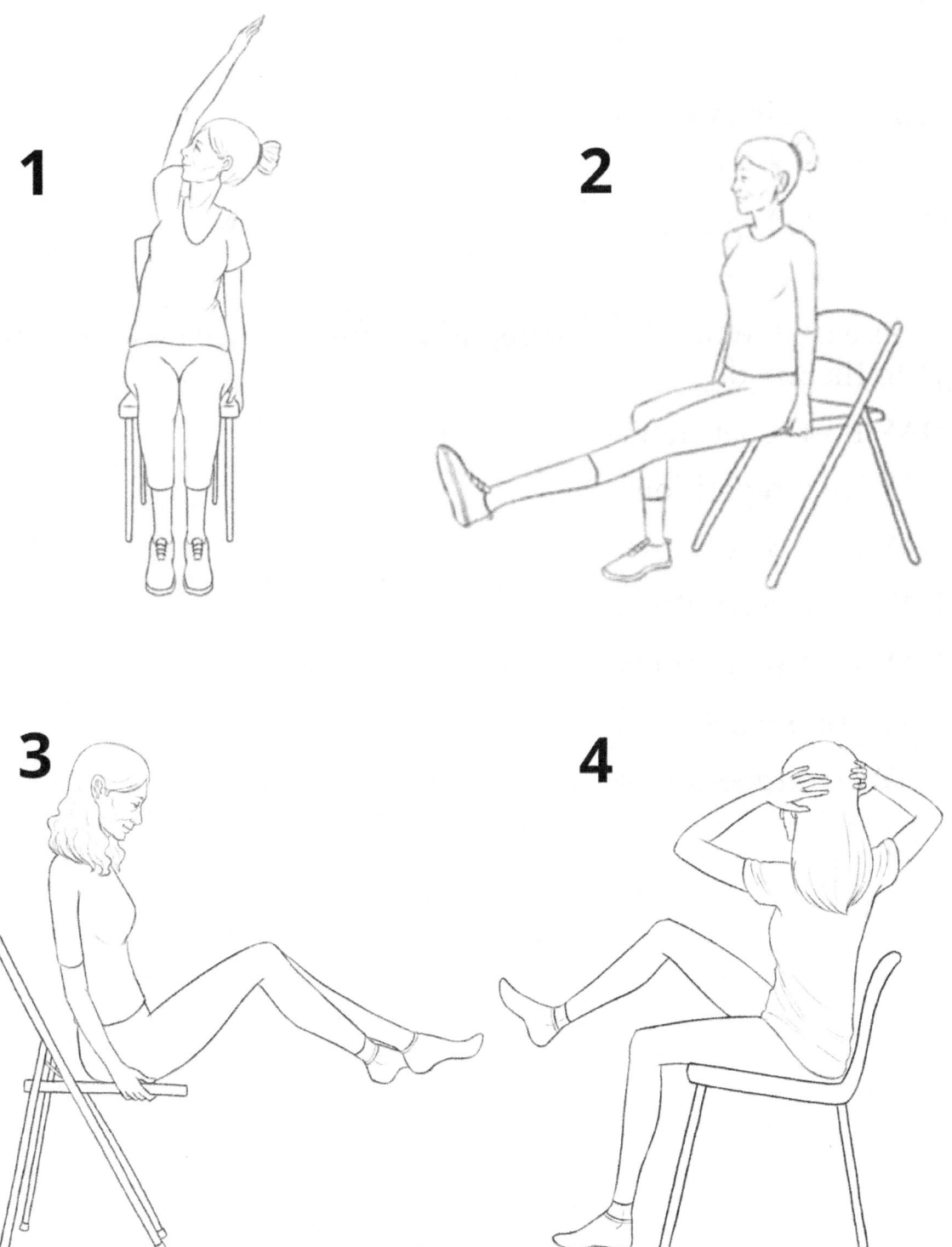

THIRD WEEK

During the third week, you will practice all the balance poses from Chapter 3:

1. Seated Tree Pose
2. Seated Chair Twist
3. Seated Warrior I
4. Chair Side Leg Lifts

Try to increase the number of repetitions for balance poses by one from the 15th to the 21st day:

- ☐ DAY 15: 1 repetition
- ☐ DAY 16: 2 repetitions
- ☐ DAY 17: 3 repetitions
- ☐ DAY 18: 4 repetitions
- ☐ DAY 19: 5 repetitions
- ☐ DAY 20: 6 repetitions
- ☐ DAY 21: 7 repetitions

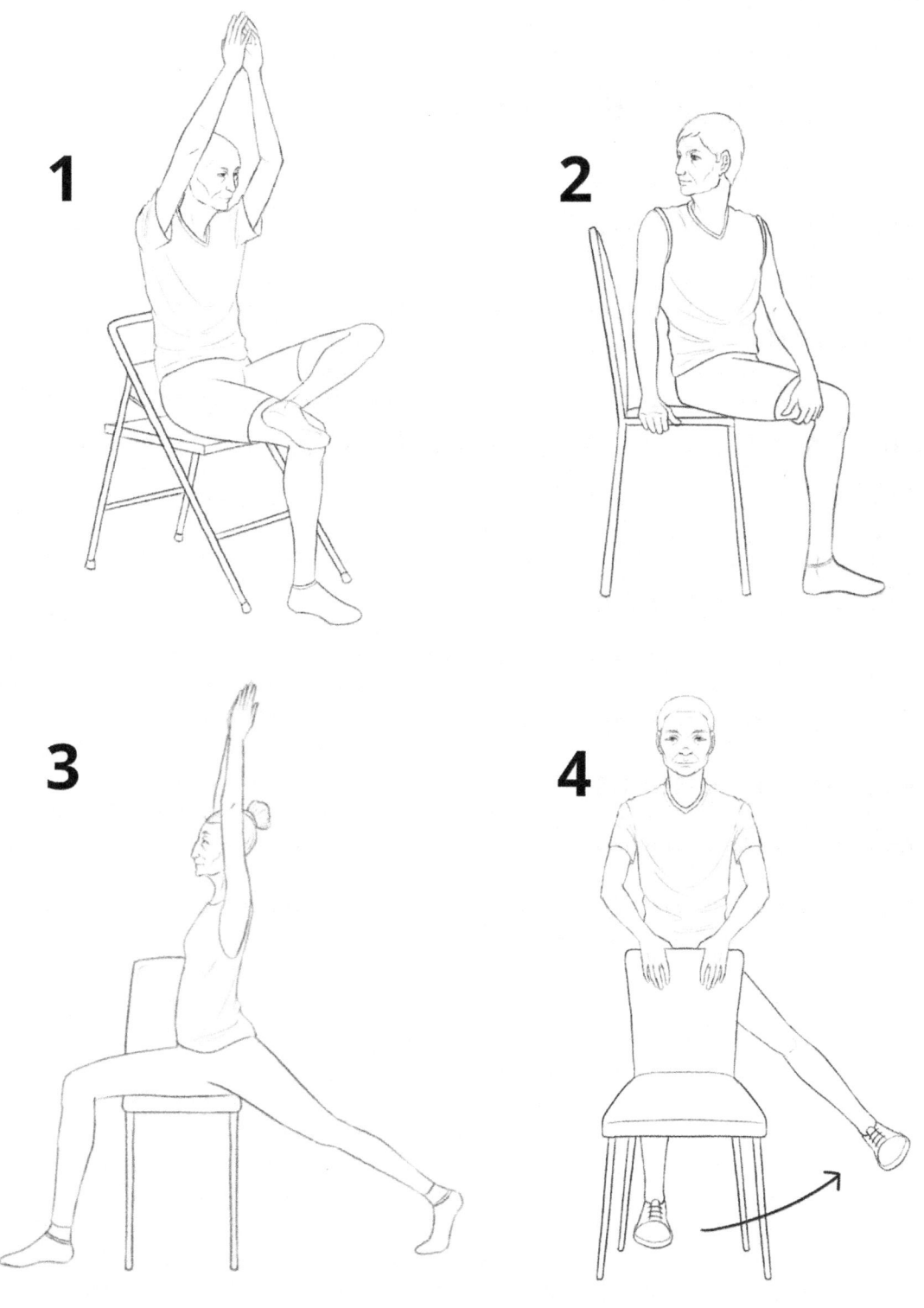

FOURTH WEEK

In the fourth week, you will practice postures related to metabolism and digestion from Chapter 3:

1. Seated High Knee March
2. Seated Diaphragmatic Breathing
3. Chair High Lunge
4. Chair Downward Dog
5. Child's Pose
6. Cobra Pose

Try to increase the number of repetitions by one from the 22nd to the 28th day:

- ☐ DAY 22: 1 repetition
- ☐ DAY 23: 2 repetitions
- ☐ DAY 24: 3 repetitions
- ☐ DAY 25: 4 repetitions
- ☐ DAY 26: 5 repetitions
- ☐ DAY 27: 6 repetitions
- ☐ DAY 28: 7 repetitions

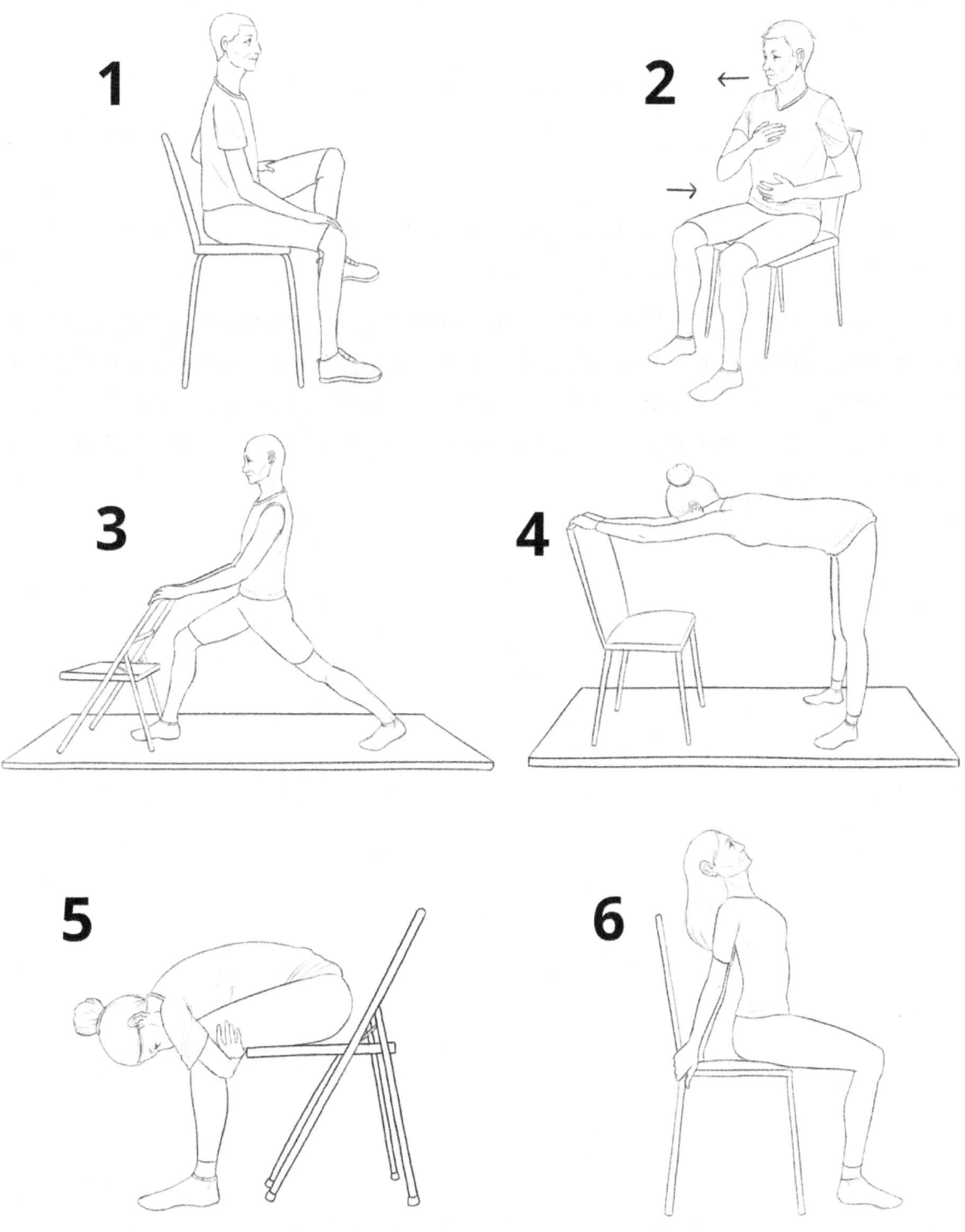

After four weeks, the activities and tips can be easily incorporated into your daily activities and chair yoga practice.

After the fourth week, you should have enough confidence and knowledge to be able to combine the poses presented in this book on your own.

Keep carrying out the activities, especially keeping a journal.

A regular journal gives you a clear insight into your progress after a few months.

I'm sure the tips and activities for the first four weeks of your chair yoga practice will keep you motivated and on track.

You can continue using this workout routine even after wrapping up the fourth week, but I would like to encourage you to incorporate best seated exercises into your workouts to supercharge your weight loss from Chapter 5 or to try the workouts from Chapter 6 "Chair Yoga in Under 10 Minutes".

CHAPTER 5: 10 Best Seated Exercises to Supercharge Your Weight Loss

"Your body is your most priceless possession; take care of it."

- Jack Lalanne

In this chapter, you will explore ten chair yoga poses that will supercharge your weight loss. Most of these poses are upgrades of poses from the previous chapters.

The poses detailed in this chapter are based on traditional yoga postures with fitness elements. These are more dynamic movements that will help you get rid of excess body weight.

You certainly have no reason to worry; it is still a gentle chair yoga practice, whose primary goal is **safety**.

In this chapter, cardio and muscle-toning yoga poses await you, the ultimate way to supercharge your weight loss.

When performing these poses, adhere to the following guidelines:

- Perform each position and movement correctly, following the detailed instructions.
- Follow the rhythm of your body as you practice the positions and movements; do not rush. That way, you will perform them safely.
- Remain fully aware of each inhale and exhale. This way, you will be fully present during your chair yoga practice. While executing these positions and movements, practice three-layer breathing (stomach, lungs, and tops of the lungs). Remember to try to make your exhalation twice as long as your inhalation.
- Stay consistent with your chair yoga practice. Practice it every day, without excuses.
- Finally, take care of your diet; start eating healthier if you haven't already.

Seated Jumping Jacks

This chair-based cardio exercise is a great way to keep yourself from feeling tired during the day.

Thanks to seated jumping jacks, you will:
- Strengthen your heart and lungs
- Improve metabolic function
- Ultimately impacting your weight loss.

Instructions, step-by-step:
- Sit in the middle of the chair with your back straight.
- Your feet are resting firmly on the yoga mat, hip width apart.
- With an inhale, stretch your arms out to the side and raise them above your head.
- With an exhalation, lower your arms to the starting position on the side of the chair.
- Do a maximum of three sets of twenty repetitions. If you can't do twenty repetitions, do the number of repetitions that your body is currently comfortable with.

During the first set, you can raise your arms very slowly; you can count to three while raising your arms. During the second set, you can count to two as you raise your arms. During the third set, you can count once while raising your hands.

This way, you improve your cardio rhythm, which positively impacts your weight loss goal.

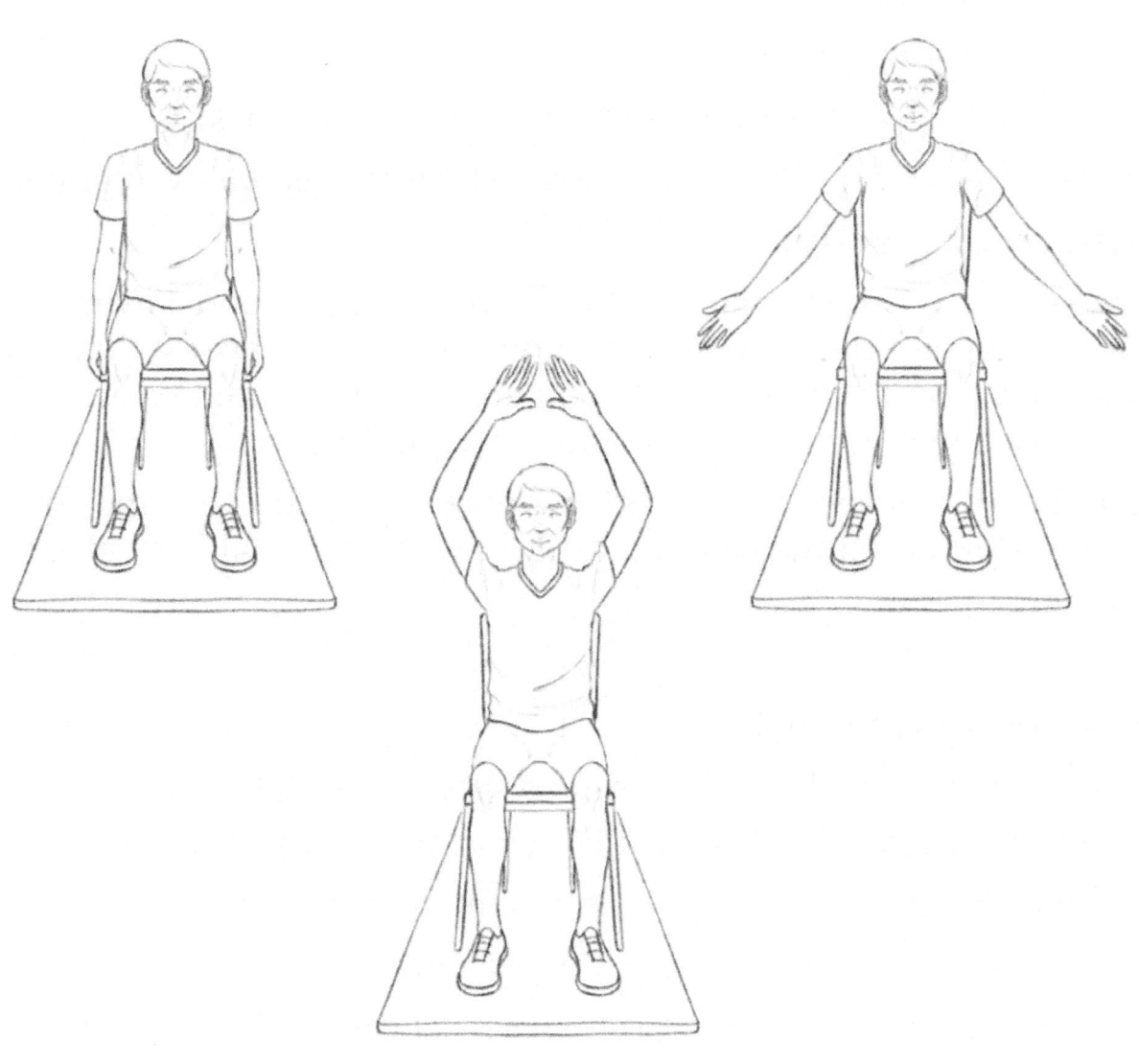

Seated Toe Taps

This move has two variations. I advise you to start by practicing the first variation. If you find that your body is ready for a slightly more demanding movement, you can practice the second variation.

Thanks to this movement, you will:
- Improve flexibility
- Strengthen your joints
- Gently stretch your calves, soles of your feet, and toes.

This is a great way to improve balance, which can lead to weight loss.

In what way exactly?

When you have strong ankles and well-stretched feet and calves, you will be more stable when practicing movements and poses that require greater balance. The more stable you are, the better and easier you will perform cardio movements that lead to weight loss.

You must always keep in mind that every pose and every movement is very important on a micro level, especially if your goal is to attain your ideal body weight.

Instructions, step-by-step:
- Sit in the middle of the chair with your back straight.
- Your feet are resting firmly on the yoga mat, hip width apart.
- Inhale and lift your toes, pointing them upwards.
- Exhaling, lower your feet onto the yoga mat.
- Repeat this movement for 3 sets. Each set can have ten repetitions.

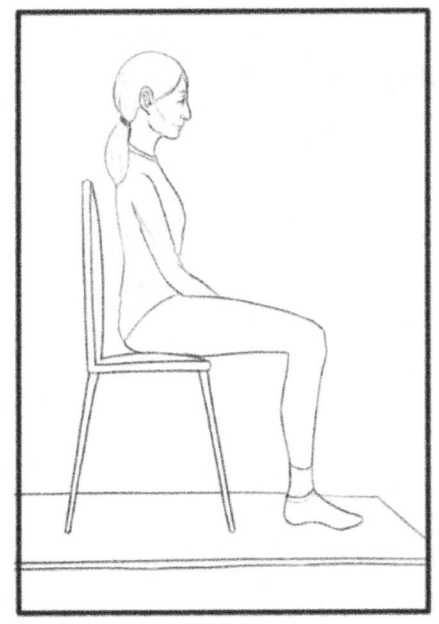 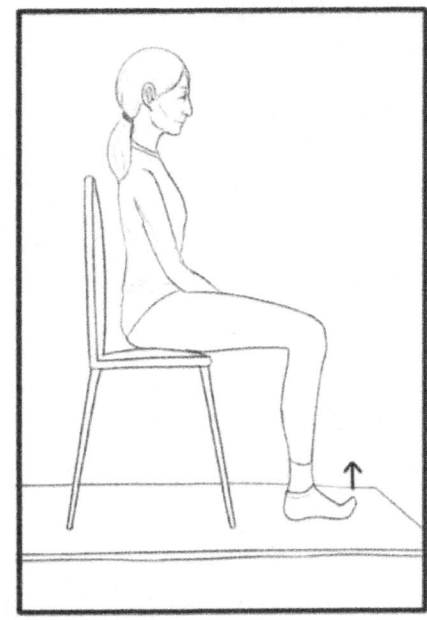

Another variation involves your legs being stretched.

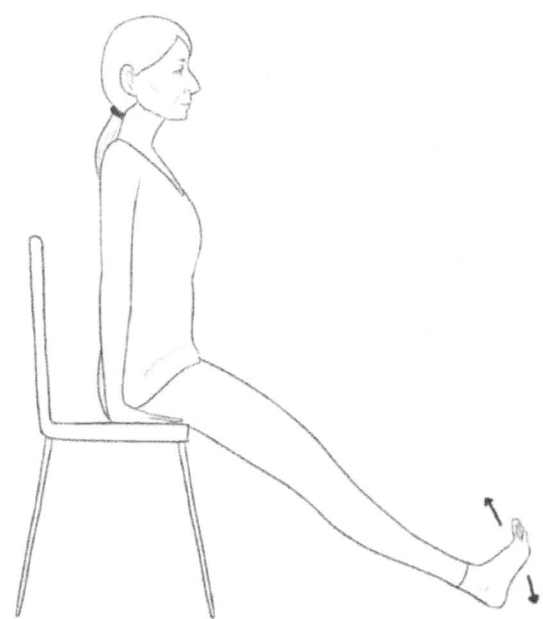

- Sit in the middle of the chair with your back straight.
- Your feet are resting firmly on the yoga mat, hip width apart.
- Stretch and extend your legs.
- As you inhale, stretch your toes toward your body.
- As you exhale, stretch your toes down.
- Repeat this movement for 3 sets. Each set can have ten repetitions.

During the first variation, you can rest your back completely on the backrest if you feel more stable during the movement.

Seated Knee to Elbow

This movement has four possible variations. The variation you choose to practice should respect your current mobility and strength.

Your current body weight also plays an important role in performing this movement. If the first variation is difficult for you, try the other variations. Evaluate them and find the ideal variation for you right now.

Thanks to this movement, you will:
- Strengthen your oblique abdominal muscles
- Strengthen your core

A strong core greatly impacts your ability to maintain correct posture.

First Variation

Instructions, step-by-step:
- Sit on a chair with your back straight. Lean your back against the back of the chair.
- Your feet are resting firmly on the yoga mat, hip width apart.
- Interlace your fingers behind your head and spread your elbows to the side. Your elbows should be in line with your shoulders. In case you feel stiffness in your neck or shoulder blades and you're unable to open your elbows so that they are in line with your shoulders, try variation number two.
- Inhale in the position; exhaling, lift your left knee and move your right elbow towards your left knee. If you can, move until your knee and elbow touch.
- During this movement, rotate your upper body towards the raised knee.
- Alternate on the left and right sides.
- Perform 10 repetitions on each side if you can. Otherwise, perform the highest number of repetitions within your limits.

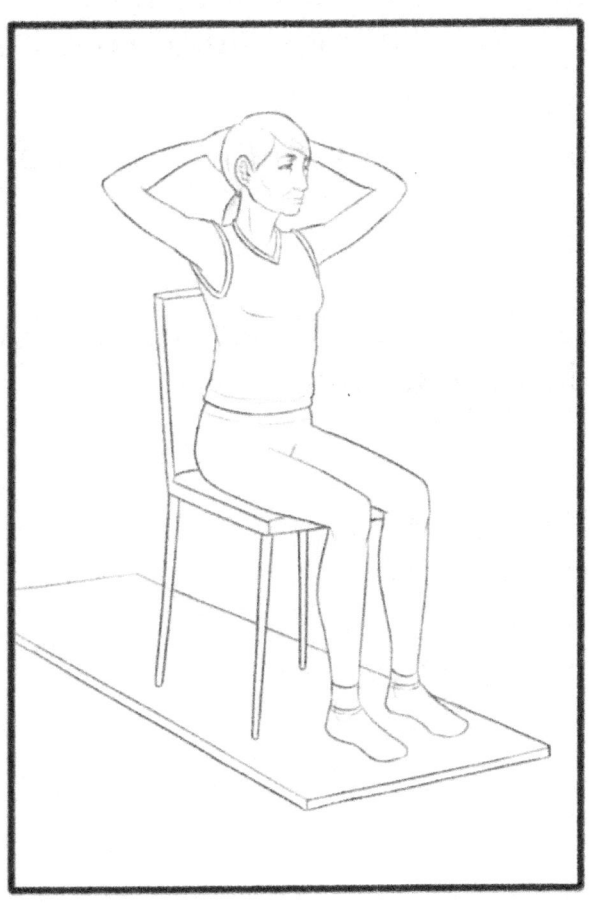 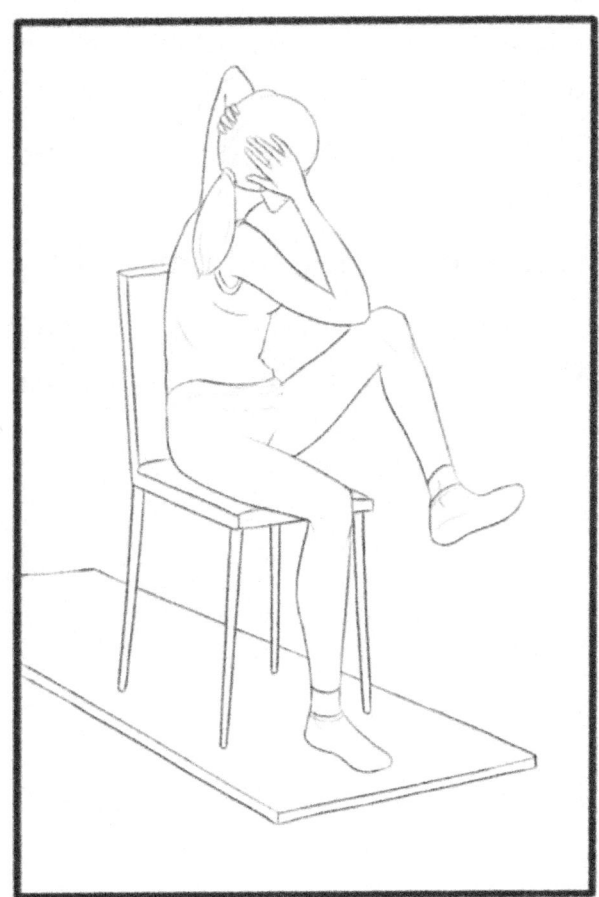

Second Variation

Instructions, step-by-step:

- Sit on a chair with your back straight. Lean against the back of the chair.
- Your feet are resting firmly on the yoga mat, hip width apart.
- In this variation, do not interlace your fingers behind your head; your hands are at the sides of your body in the initial position. However, there is still rotation of the upper body towards the raised knee.
- Inhale in the position; exhaling, lift your left knee and move your right elbow towards your left knee. If you can, move until your knee and elbow touch.
- During this movement, rotate your upper body towards the raised knee.
- Alternate on the left and right sides.
- Perform 10 repetitions on each side if you can. Otherwise, perform the highest number of repetitions within your limits.

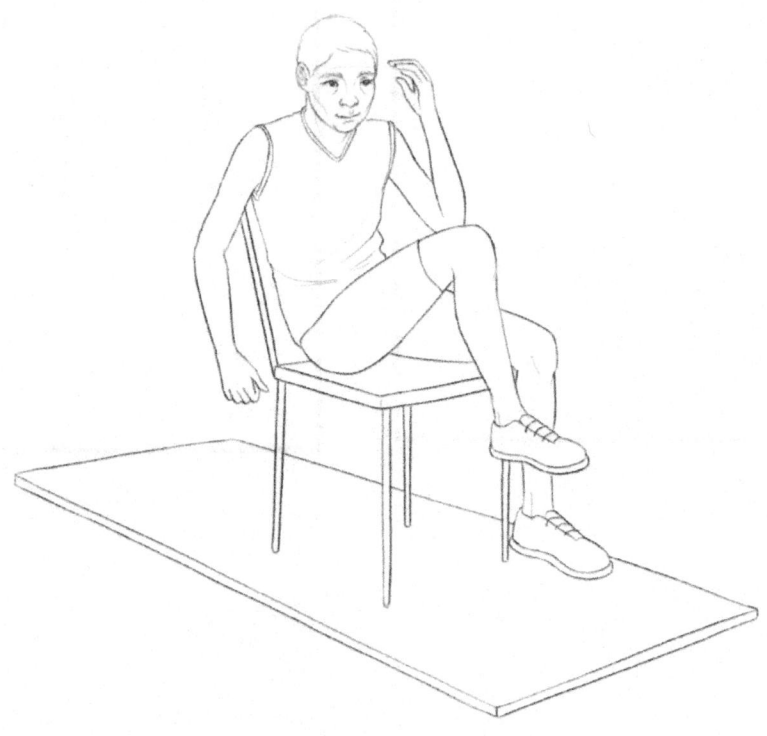

Third Variation

Instructions, step-by-step:

If you find it challenging to perform upper body rotations, try the third or fourth variation.

- Sit on a chair with your back straight. Lean your back against the back of the chair.
- Your feet are resting firmly on the yoga mat, hip width apart.
- In this variation, do not interlace your fingers behind your head. Raise your right arm above your head while the other is at your side.
- Inhale in the position; exhaling, lift your left knee and move your right elbow towards your left knee. If you can, move until your knee and elbow touch.
- During this movement, do not rotate your upper body towards the raised knee.
- Work alternately on the left and right sides.
- Perform 10 repetitions on each side if you can. Otherwise, perform the highest number of repetitions within your limits.

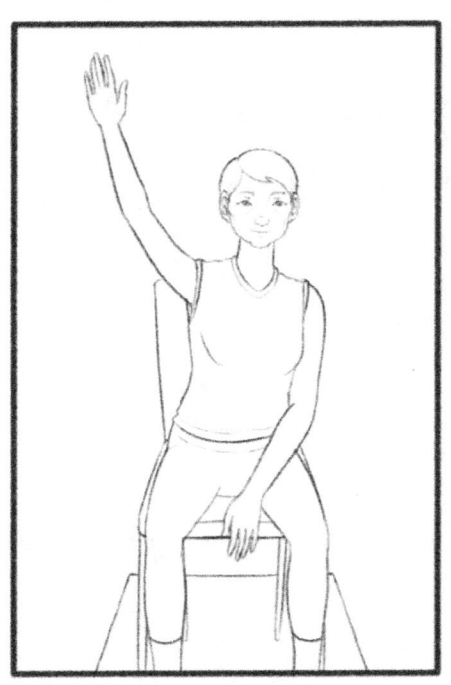 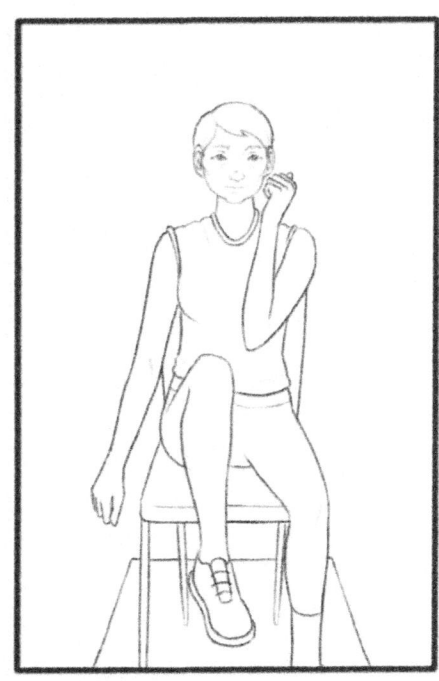

Fourth Variation

Instructions, step-by-step:

- Sit on a chair with your back straight. Lean your back against the back of the chair.
- Your feet are resting firmly on the yoga mat, hip width apart.
- In this variation, interlace your fingers behind your head while your elbows are in front of your body, in line with your shoulders.
- Inhale in the position, and as you exhale, slowly lower your upper body towards your thighs.
- If you can, lower your elbows to your knees.
- Perform 10 repetitions on each side if you can. Otherwise, perform the highest number of repetitions within your limits.

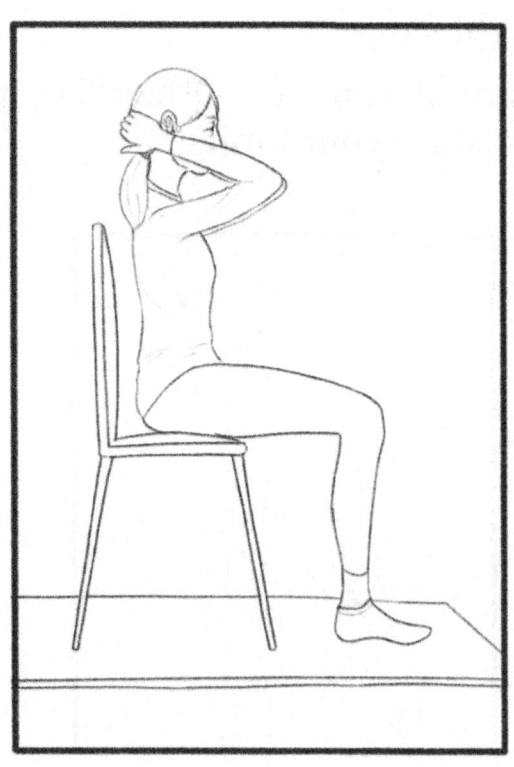
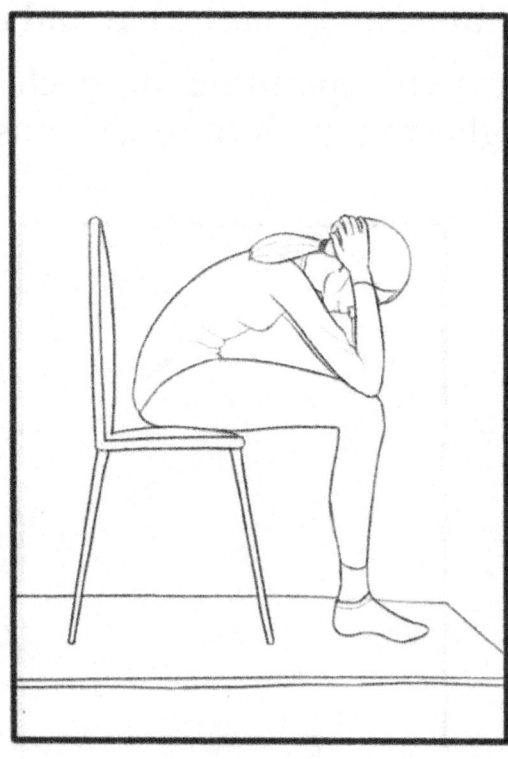

Seated Cat-Cow Stretch - dynamic version

You've been introduced to this movement before; however, there is one small modification that makes this movement more dynamic.

By performing this movement, you'll:

- Strengthen your abdominal and lower back muscles
- Gently stretch your back and neck
- Open your chest

Instructions, step-by-step:

- Sit at the center of the chair with your back straight.
- Your feet are resting firmly on the yoga mat, hip width apart.
- Inhale in the position and stretch your back upwards as much as you can.
- Your chin is level with your chest, your arms are outstretched, and your palms are on your knees.
- Exhaling, bend in the upper part of the back and go with the chin towards the sternum. Your arms remain stretched; do not bend them at the elbows.
- An important difference from the same movement presented before is the way you breathe. During this movement, the exhalation is not twice as long as the inhalation. It involves very fast inhalations and exhalations; therefore, the movement itself is much faster. Try to make each inhalation and exhalation one second long.
- Perform 10 repetitions if you can. Otherwise, perform the highest number of repetitions within your limits.

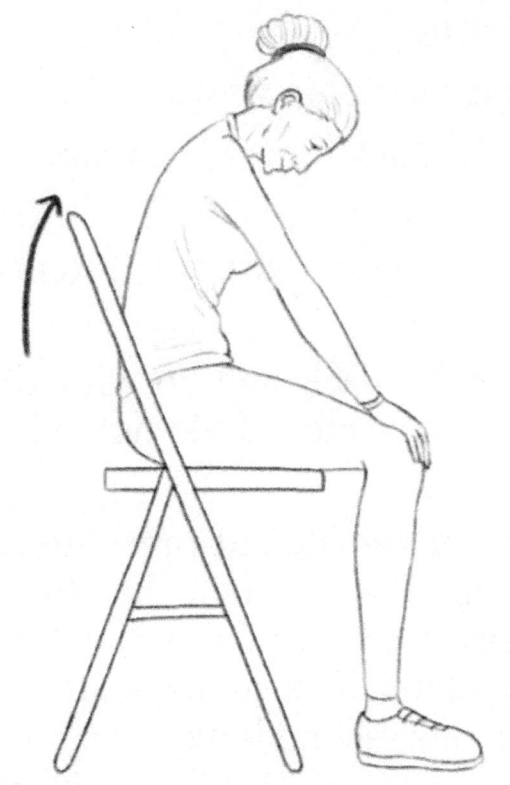
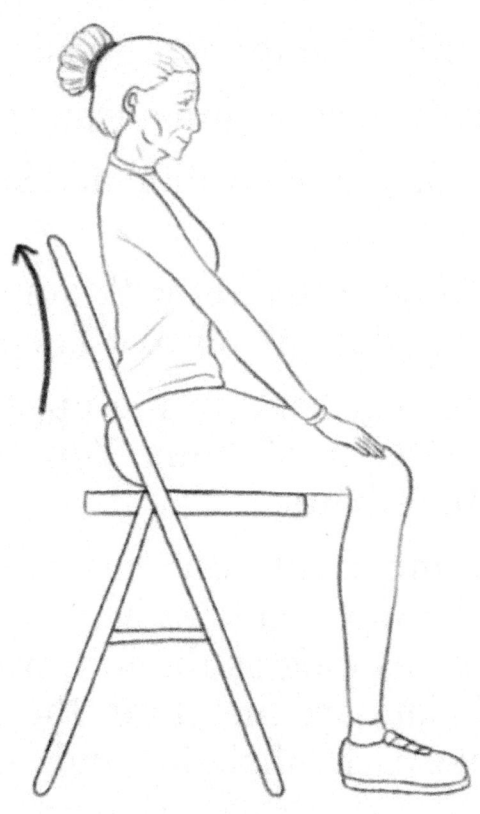

78

Seated Shoulder Shrug

This movement will:

- Improve the mobility of your shoulder blades
- Improve the mobility of your shoulders
- Relieve accumulated stress in the shoulders and neck

When you are exposed to stress for a long period of time, it can cause weight gain. Consequently, when you get rid of stress, you are also working on weight loss.

This movement has two variations; you can practice one or both.

First Variation

Instructions, step-by-step:

- Sit at the center of the chair with your back straight.
- Your feet are resting firmly on the yoga mat, hip width apart.
- You can place your palms on your thighs. Your chin is level with your chest.
- With an inhale, lift your shoulders up toward your ears.
- Exhaling, lower your shoulders down to the starting position.
- If you can, repeat this movement between 10 and 20 times, otherwise perform the number of repetitions within your limits.

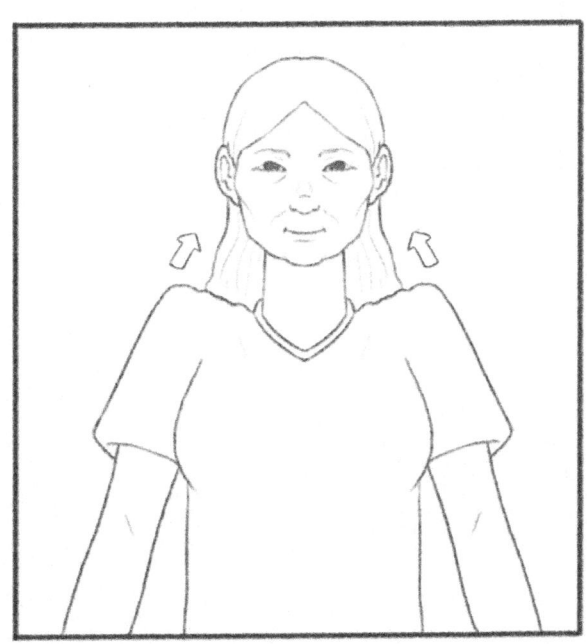

Second Variation

Instructions, step-by-step:

- Sit at the center of the chair with your back straight.
- Your feet are resting firmly on the yoga mat, hip width apart.
- You can place your palms on your thighs. Your chin is level with your chest.
- Breathing with a rhythm that suits you, alternately raise and lower your left and right shoulder. When you raise your left shoulder, lower your right shoulder.
- Perform this movement between 10 and 20 times if you can. Otherwise, perform the number of repetitions within your limits.

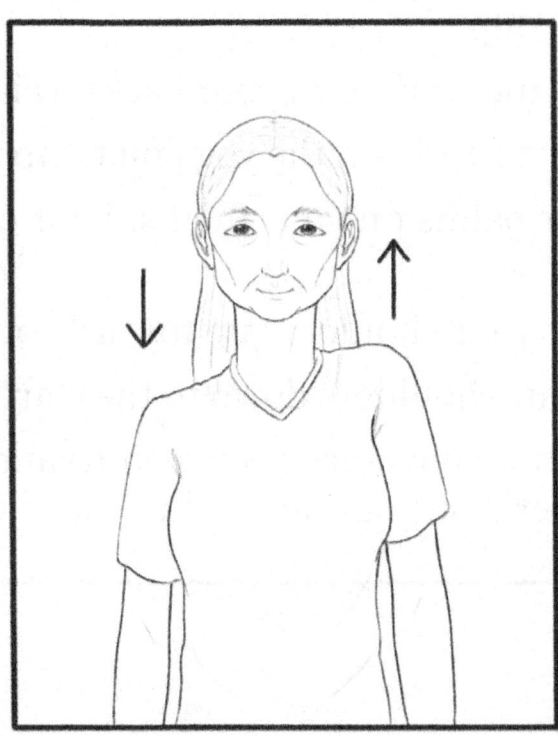

Seated Leg Circles

This movement resembles a leg extension, but one element is added that makes it more dynamic.

With this movement, you will:
- Increase the mobility of your lower legs
- Strengthen your quadriceps
- Work on the micro level to open your hips and pelvis

Instructions, step-by-step:
- Sit on the front part of the chair with your back straight. Hold on to the sides of the seat for stability.
- Your feet are hip width apart on the yoga mat.
- Inhale in the position, and as you exhale, lift your right leg as far as you can. If you can, stretch it fully forward.
- Extend the toes of the right foot further forward if your body allows. In this way, you will stretch the calf and hamstrings of the right leg.
- Make between five and ten circles, first to the left, then to the right.
- Return the right leg to the starting position.
- Repeat for the left leg.

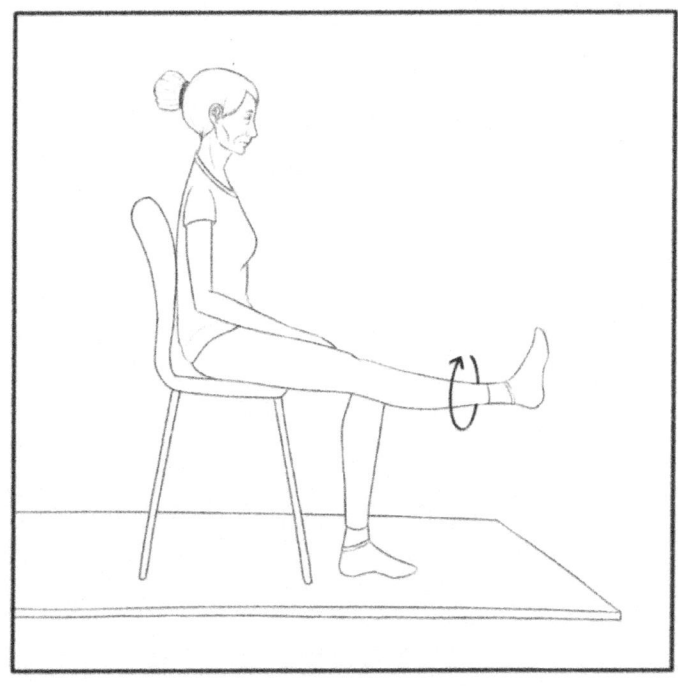

Reverse Crunches

This movement may seem simple to you, but you will notice that it is very challenging, primarily because both legs are raised at the same time and bent at the knees.

This movement engages:

- The abdominal muscles
- Legs
- Upper body muscles

The more stable your upper body, the easier it will be to perform this movement.

Instructions, step-by-step:

- Sit on a chair, resting your back on the backrest, and hold the side of the chair with your hands. Your back is completely straightened.
- Your feet are together on the yoga mat.
- Inhale in the position; exhaling, bend both legs at the knees and raise them as close to the body as possible. Bring your thighs into contact with your chest if you can.
- Inhale and return your legs to the starting position.
- Perform 5 to 10 repetitions.

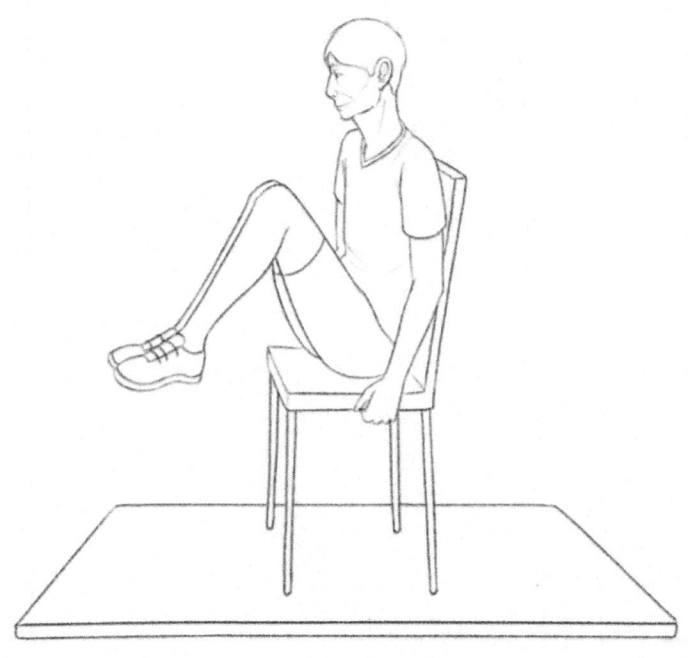

Seated Knee Head

This movement:
- Engages the core
- opens the midsection
- Improves digestive function

Instructions, step-by-step:
- Sit on a chair, resting your back on the backrest. Your hands can be at your sides. Your back is completely straight.
- Your feet are hip width apart on the yoga mat.
- Inhale in the position; exhaling, lift and bend the right leg at the knee. Wrap your arms around it and bring your head as close to the knee as possible. Connect your head and knee if you can.
- Inhale and return the leg to the starting position.
- Repeat on the left side.
- Alternately, perform 5 to 10 repetitions for each leg.

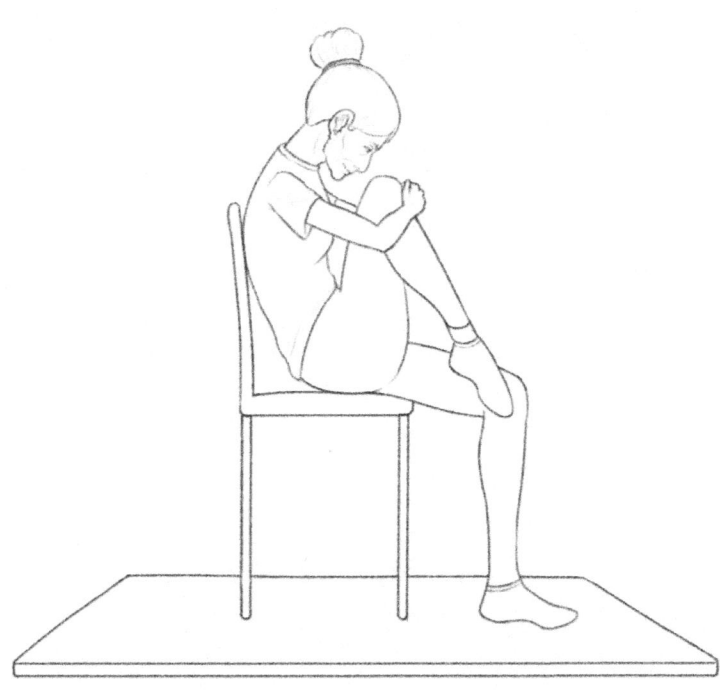

Seated Mountain Climbers

This movement activates:
- Muscles in the lower body
- Muscles in the upper body

While performing this movement, breathe with your own rhythm. It is important to remain aware of each movement; don't rush.

Instructions, step-by-step:
- Sit at the center of the chair with your back straight.
- Your feet are hip width apart on the yoga mat.
- Start breathing to your rhythm.
- While raising your right arm above your head, lift your left leg up, bent at the knee. Then lower your right arm and left leg, lift your left arm and right leg.
- Do this movement five to ten times.

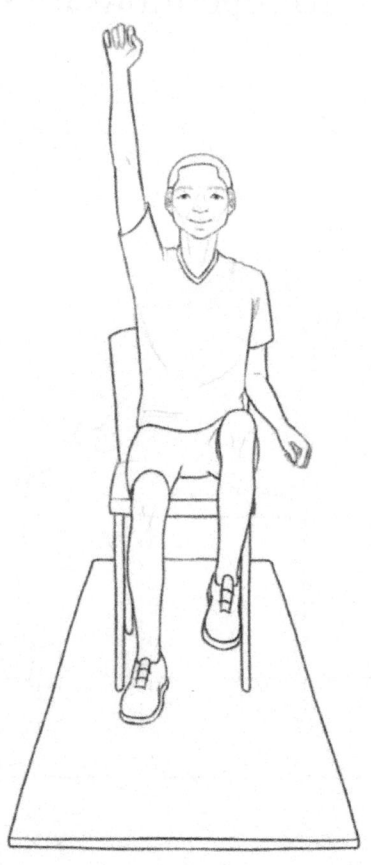

Seated Mindful Breathing

This breathing technique will allow you to:

- Become aware of the present moment
- Relieve accumulated stress and anxiety
- Establish proper metabolic function - which will ultimately help you in attaining your ideal body weight

Instructions, step-by-step:

- Sit at the center of the chair with your back straight.
- Your feet are hip width apart on the yoga mat.
- Close your eyes and start breathing to your rhythm.
- Do not pay attention to the length of inhalation and exhalation at first.
- After a few minutes of breathing in your rhythm, exhale so that your exhalation is so long that you can count to four.
- Don't breathe until you count to four.
- Inhale to the count of four.
- Hold your breath for a count of four.
- Exhale to the count of four.
- Repeat this breathing pattern for the next 2 to 3 minutes.

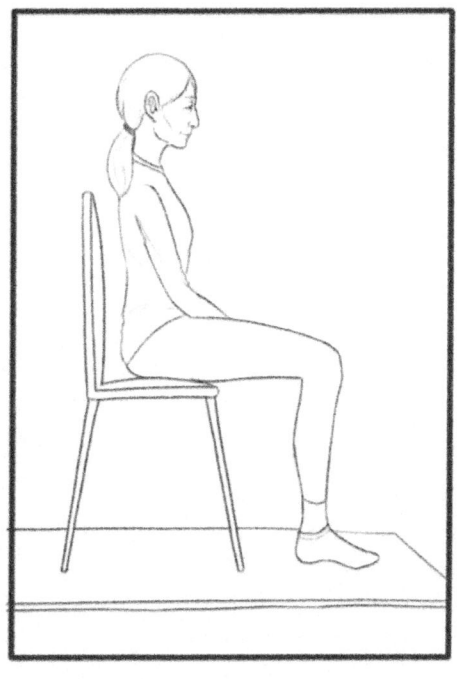

In this chapter, you were introduced to movements that will impact your weight loss if you include them in your regular chair yoga practice.

Given the number of variations that exist within each movement, you are free to practice the movements, ensuring to respect your current physical capabilities.

In the next chapter, you will be given the opportunity to combine the poses and movements into one effective and fast workout.

In this way, you will be better equipped to achieve your weight loss goal.

CHAPTER 6:
Chair Yoga in Under 10 Minutes

"The way we spend our time defines who we are."

- Jonathan Estrin

In this chapter, you will explore two different workouts whose main characteristic is their effectiveness and the time it takes to perform them. The first workout is intended for people who are just beginning their chair yoga practice or simply have not yet developed the appropriate flexibility and mobility of the body.

If you belong to that category, it is important to practice the first workout until you develop the appropriate mobility and flexibility in your body.

What is meant by appropriate flexibility and mobility of the body?

This includes movements that you can practice in workout 2 without straining or limiting the range of motion of your arms, legs, and upper and lower body.

Until you establish the appropriate flexibility and mobility in your body, I recommend you do workout 1.

The first part of the workout is intended for beginners, while the second part of the workout is intended for those at an intermediate level.

The workout emphasizes exactly where the beginner level ends and where the intermediate part begins.

TIP: The third part of the workout is focused on relaxation. It is very important to do relaxation after each workout. It's important not to miss it, regardless of the part of the workout you do.

The second workout is intended for exercisers whose flexibility and mobility are more developed; that is, they do not experience extensive limitations in range of motion or possible pain.

Each workout is designed to last less than ten minutes. In the beginning, you may need a little more than ten minutes to perform them, but as you become more familiar with the instructions, you'll execute the entire workout in less time with minimal issues.

Each workout consists of three parts:

- Introductory positions whose main goal is to warm up your body. This will help properly lubricate your joints, relax your muscles, and eliminate any feeling of stiffness in your body.
- These positions are followed by cardio movements (which we covered in the previous chapter).
- At the end of each workout, there will be positions aimed at relaxing your body.

After a while, you can start combining the poses and movements to create your own sequence, which can last longer than ten minutes.

Before personalizing the workout, perform each workout in this chapter several times (at least once a week), primarily because each workout is designed to help you progress in a safe and simple way to attain your desired body weight.

Workout #1 - beginner (and intermediate) level

TIP: From first to sixth position is the beginner level. Be sure to do the last part of the workout (mindful breathing) when you do the beginner level.

1st part - Beginner level exercises

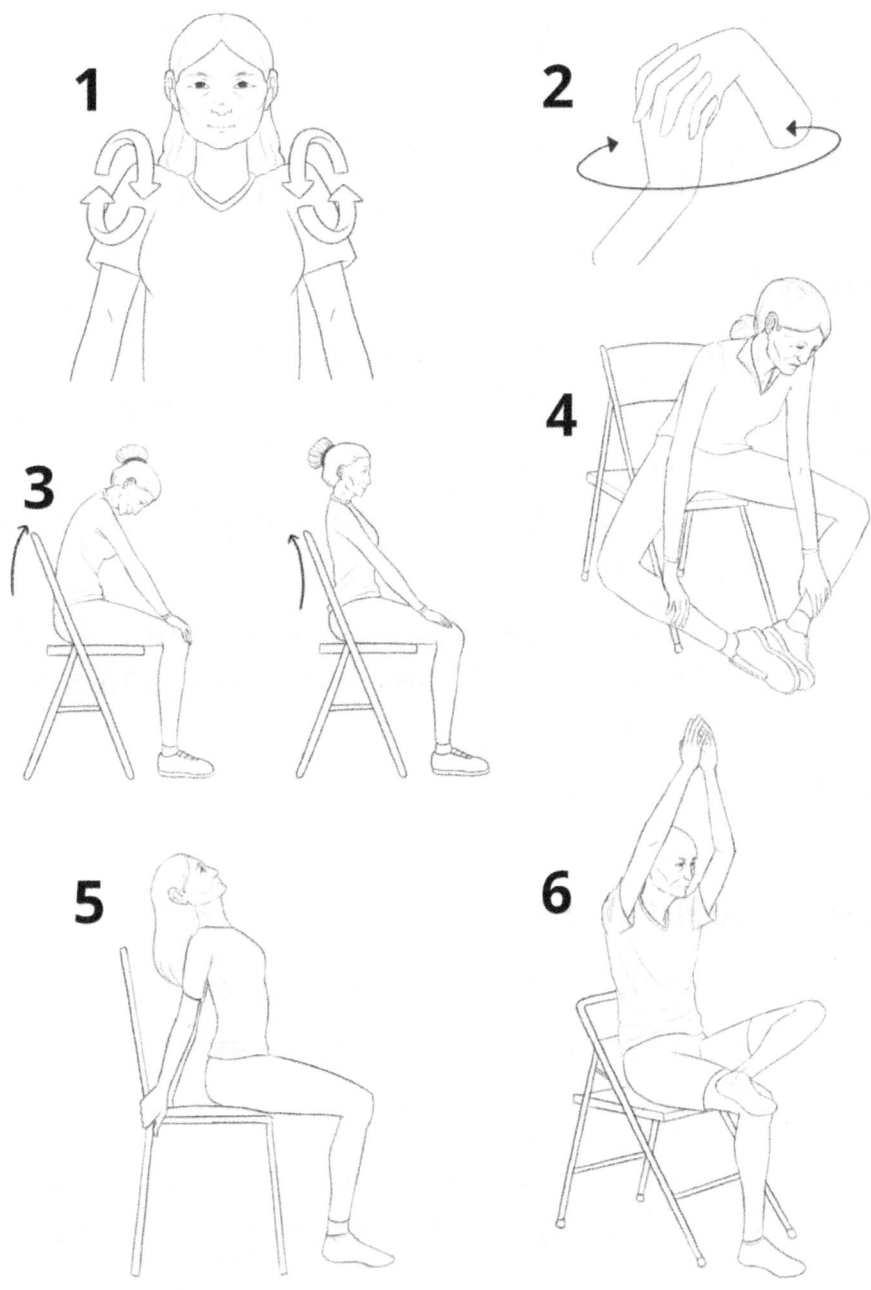

1. Shoulder circles
- While sitting with your back straight on a chair, make five to ten circles with your shoulders, first forward, then backward.
- During this movement, breathe in three layers.

2. Rotation of the wrists
- Sitting with your back straight, raise your arms to chest height and interlace your fingers.
- Do ten circles; first to the right, then to the left.

3. Cat cow pose
- Sit on the chair with your feet firmly positioned hip width apart on the yoga mat and your palms on your knees (your arms are outstretched).
- Exhaling, lower your head and chin towards your sternum, creating a curve in your upper back.
- Inhaling, lift your head and chin back to the starting position, expanding your chest forward. Your back will gently stretch as you inhale.
- Repeat five times.

4. Seated Butterfly Stretch
- Sit on the edge of the chair with your back straight.
- Put your heels together and if you can, put your feet and toes together.
- Move your knees to the side as far as you can.
- When you can no longer bring your knees down to the side, lower your upper body and grasp your feet, ankles, or calves with your hands.
- From that position, if your body allows, move your knees down to the side a little more. This gently opens your hips and inner thighs.
- Stay in the position for 5 breaths.

- Inhale and return to the starting position.

5. Cobra Pose

- Sit at the center of the chair with your back straight and your feet hip-width apart.
- Stretch your arms back, gripping the bottom of the chair back.
- With an inhale, expand the chest forward and move your head back if you are comfortable. If not, then don't stretch your neck back.
- Exhaling, return to the starting position.
- Repeat this movement 5 to 10 times.

6. Seated Tree Pose

- Sit on a chair with your back straight. Your feet are firmly on the yoga mat, about hip-width apart. If you want, rest your back on the back of the chair.
- Lift your right foot and place it on your left knee. If you find it challenging, lower your foot to the inside of your left thigh. If you find that challenging, place your right foot on your left ankle.
- Hold on to the sides of the chair with both hands.
- If you feel you have a good balance, you can try to do a full pose. Stretch your arms above your head and bring your palms together.
- Stay in the selected position for 5 breaths.
- Repeat on the other side.

2nd part - Intermediate level exercises

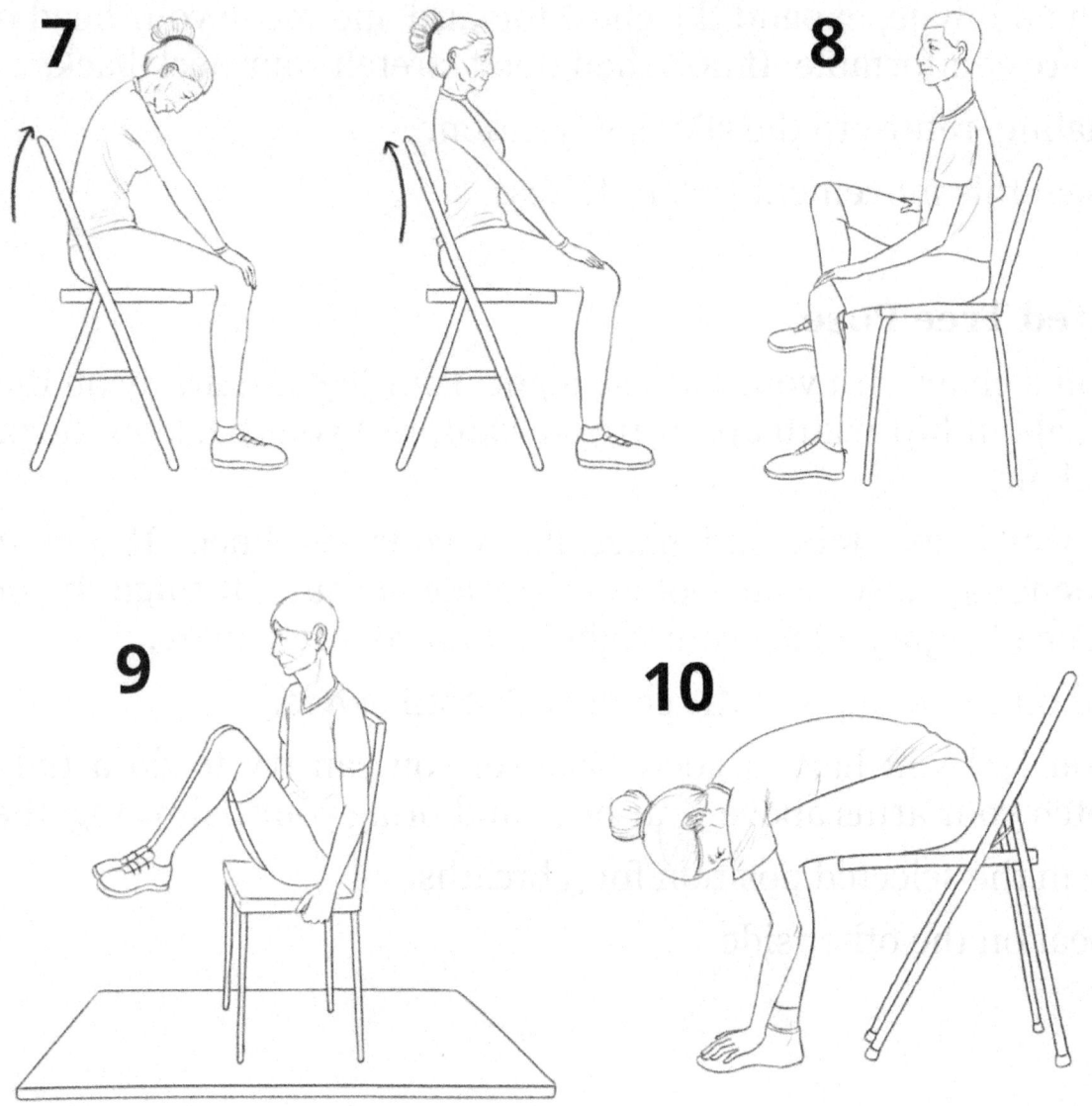

7. Seated Cat-Cow Stretch - dynamic version

- Sit at the center of the chair with your back straight.
- Your feet are resting firmly on the yoga mat, hip width apart.
- Inhale in the position and stretch your back upwards as much as you can.
- Your chin is level with your chest, your arms are outstretched, and your palms are on your knees.
- Exhaling, bend in the upper part of the back and lower your chin towards your sternum. Your arms remain stretched; do not bend them at the elbows.
- An important difference from the same movement practiced before is the breathing style. During this movement, the exhalation is not twice as long as the inhalation. It involves very fast inhalations and exhalations; therefore, the movement is much faster. Try to make each inhalation and exhalation one second long.
- If you can, perform 10 repetitions. Otherwise perform the number of repetitions within your limits.

8. Seated High Knee March

- Sit on a chair with your back straight. Your feet are placed hip-width apart on the yoga mat.
- Hold on to the sides of the chair with both hands.
- Inhale in the position; as you exhale, lift your right leg towards your chest, bending it at the knee. Inhale, then lower the foot to the starting position.
- Do it for the left leg.
- Repeat this movement alternately 5 to 10 times.

9. Reverse Crunches

- Sit on a chair, resting your back on the backrest, and hold the side of the chair with your hands. Keep your back straight.
- Your feet are together on the yoga mat.
- Inhale in the position; exhaling, bend both legs at the knees and raise them as close to the body as possible. Bring your thighs into contact with your chest if you can.
- Inhale and return your legs to the starting position.
- Perform 5 to 10 repetitions.

10. Seated Forward Bend

- Sit on the edge of a chair with your back straight and your feet firmly planted hip-width apart on the yoga mat.
- Inhale in the position, and with an exhale without moving your hips, lower your upper body down towards your thighs.
- If your body allows it, bring your upper body into contact with your thighs. If you are unable to, stop in a position that is comfortable for you; don't force your whole body.
- To gently stretch your back and groin, wrap your arms around your knees, linking your hands at your shins.
- Stay in that position, breathing in three layers for five inhalations and exhalations.
- After that, take a breath and slowly return to the starting position.

3rd part – Relaxation

11. Seated Mindful Breathing

- Sit at the center of the chair with your back straight.
- Your feet are hip width apart on the yoga mat.
- Close your eyes and start breathing to your rhythm.
- Do not pay attention to the length of inhalation and exhalation at first.
- After a few minutes of breathing in your rhythm, exhale so that your exhalation is so long that you can count to four.
- Don't breathe until you count to four.
- Inhale to the count of four.
- Hold your breath for a count of four.
- Exhale to the count of four.
- Repeat this breathing pattern for the next 2 minutes.

Workout #2 - advanced level

1st part – Warm-up exercises

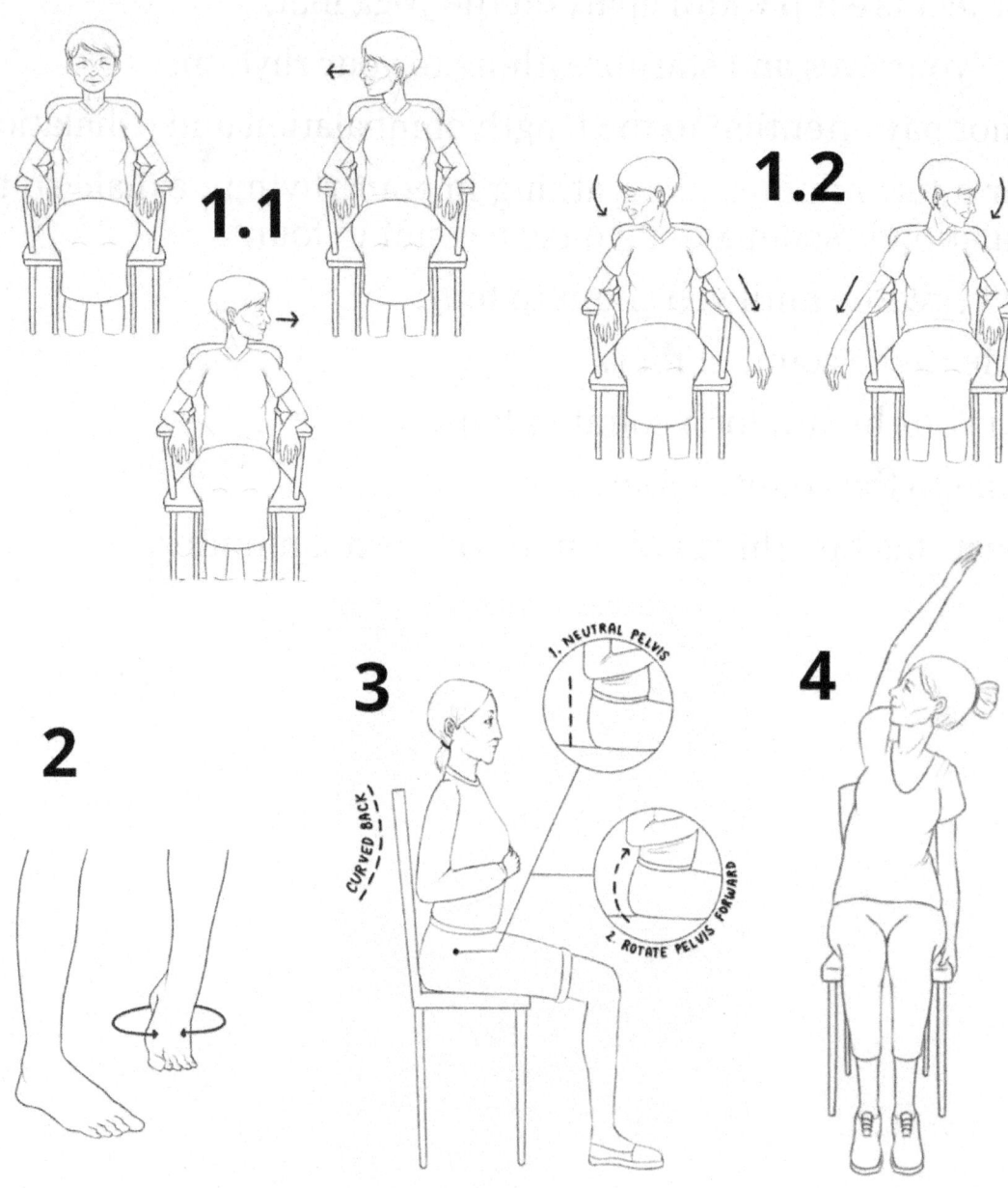

1. Neck stretches

- Sit in a chair with your back completely straight and breathe through your belly.
- The first movement involves turning your head to the right and pointing your chin towards your right shoulder. Stay in this position for five inhalations and exhalations.
- Repeat on the left side.
- The second movement involves stretching your left arm down while leaning your right ear towards your right shoulder. Stay in this position for five inhalations and exhalations.
- Repeat on the left side.
- The third movement involves moving your chin towards your breastbone. Touch your chin to your sternum if you can. This way, you stretch the back of your neck. Stay for five inhales and exhales.

2. Rotations of the toes

- While sitting with your back straight in a chair, lift your right foot off the yoga mat and do five to ten circles, first inwards, then outwards.
- After completing the circles, place your right foot on the yoga mat and lift your left foot. Repeat the same number of circles.
- During these movements, breathe in three layers.

3. Pelvic tilt

- While performing this movement, sit with your back straight, your feet firmly planted on the yoga mat, hip width apart.
- To remain aware of the movement, place your palms on your stomach.
- As you inhale, your pelvis will move forward, and as you exhale, it will move backwards.
- During this movement, breathe with your stomach. That's why I recommend placing your palms on your stomach.
- Do ten forward and backward pelvic movements.

4. Seated Side Stretch

- Sit on a chair with your back straight. You can lean your back against the back of the chair if that's more convenient.
- Your feet are placed firmly on the yoga mat, your feet and knees together.
- With an inhale, raise your right arm above your body and stretch it as high as you can towards the ceiling.
- For more stability while performing this position, you can grab the seat of the chair with your left hand.
- Stay in this position for 3 to 5 breaths.
- Be aware of the stretch along the right waist and the fine extension of the right hip.
- Activate your core during the pose.
- Repeat the same movement on the left side.

2nd part – Cardio exercises

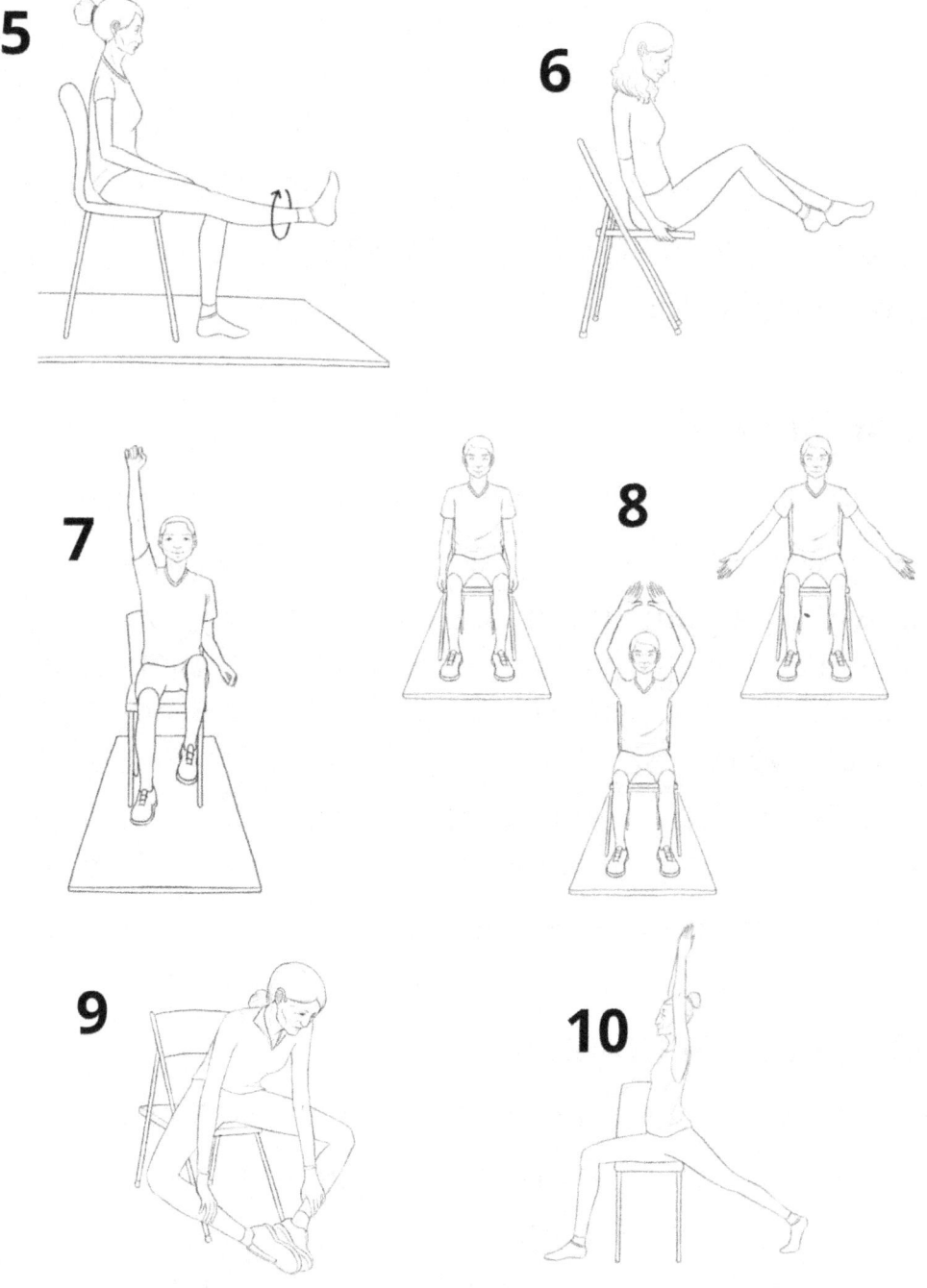

5. Seated Leg Circles

- Sit on the front part of the chair seat and support the side of the chair with your hands. Your back is completely straight.
- Your feet are hip width apart on the yoga mat.
- Inhale in the position, and as you exhale, lift your right leg up as far as you can. If you can, stretch it fully forward.
- Extend the toes of the right foot further forward if your body allows. In this way, you will stretch the calf and hamstrings of the right leg.
- Make between five and ten circles, first to the left, then to the right.
- Return the right leg to the starting position.
- Repeat on the left side.

6. Seated Boat Pose

- Sit at the center of the chair with your feet on the yoga mat.
- Grab both sides of the chair firmly with your hands.
- Very slowly lean your upper body back, all within the limits of your body. It is important that you are stable in your position. If you feel that you are losing support and stability, it is a sign that you have leaned back too far.
- Inhale in the position, and exhaling, gently lift your legs off the yoga mat as far as you can. Engage your core as you lift your legs.
- Stay in the position for 3 to 5 breaths.

7. Seated Mountain Climbers

- Sit at the center of the chair with your back straight.
- Your feet are hip width apart on the yoga mat.
- Start breathing to your rhythm.
- While raising your right arm above your head, lift your left leg, bent at the knee. Lower your right arm and left leg and lift your left arm and right leg.
- Do this movement five to ten times.

8. Seated Jumping Jacks

- Sit in the middle of the chair with your back straight.
- Your feet are resting firmly on the yoga mat, hip width apart.
- With an inhale, stretch your arms out to the side and raise them above your head.
- Exhaling, lower your arms to the starting position on the side of the chair.
- Do a maximum of three sets of twenty repetitions. If you can't do twenty repetitions, execute the number of repetitions that your body is currently comfortable with.

9. Seated Pigeon Pose

- Sit at the front of the chair with your back straight. Both of your feet are firmly on the yoga mat, about hip-width apart.
- Lift your right foot and place it on your left knee. If you cannot lift your right foot high enough, lift it as far as your body will allow, holding the right foot with your left palm.
- In both variations, place your right palm on your right knee.
- Slightly push your right knee down with your right palm, all within the limits of your body's comfort. This way, you stretch your right hip and gluteus.
- Stay in the position for 3 to 5 breaths.
- Inhale and return to the starting position by placing your right foot on the yoga mat.
- Repeat on the left side.

10. Seated Warrior I

- Sit with your back straight on a chair and your feet hip-width apart on the yoga mat.
- Rotate the left foot ninety degrees to the left. If you can't rotate your foot that far, rotate it as far as your body will allow.
- Rotate your upper body to the left.

- Stretch the right leg back and lift the right heel off the mat.
- Stretch your arms above your head and bring your palms together.
- Stay in the position for 3 to 5 breaths.
- Repeat the position on the right side.

3rd part – Relaxation

11. Sound S breathing: relaxation of the nervous system

- Sit on the chair with your back straight.
- You can slightly tilt your chin toward your breastbone. There is no need to touch the sternum.
- Take a deep breath through your nose.
- After inhaling, exhale with a sound S through the mouth, resting the tip of the tongue on the front inside of the upper teeth.
- Exhale the audible S for as long as you can.
- Repeat the breathing at least three times.

It is very important to include your chair yoga practice in your daily activities, especially if you spend most of the day sitting or are currently facing limited mobility.

You can incorporate your chair yoga practice into your daily lifestyle in the following ways:

- Morning practice.
- Regular stretching while working at the computer (stretching for 2 to 3 minutes at least every 50 minutes).
- Maintain the correct body posture (straighten your back if you notice that you have slouched, especially while working on the computer).
- Eat mindfully (chew long enough to turn food into mush).
- While watching TV, try to do some simple postures; trust me, they will be more comfortable for you.
- Practice evening stretching (a few minutes) before going to bed.
- Apply the mindfulness technique of gratitude.

In this chapter, you were introduced to two different workouts. I advise you to do each a minimum of five times before you start designing your sequences.

In this way, your body will become aware of all movements and you will be able to create your sequences in a much easier way.

It is important to emphasize that you should practice the variations that honor your current body limitations. In this way, you will stay safe and practice chair yoga long term.

At the end of this chapter, I drew your attention to the ways in which you can incorporate your chair yoga practice into your daily activities.

In the next chapter, you will understand the facts that will show you how your chair yoga practice can affect aging, stress, mindful eating, relaxation, etc.

CHAPTER 7:
Chair Yoga Beyond Exercises: Stress Reduction and Mindful Eating

"The best investment you can ever make is in your own health."

- **Unknown**

Thanks to the very gentle movements that you will practice during your chair yoga practice, as well as the breathing techniques that you will apply to relax your nervous system, chair yoga is an excellent choice to help you relax, physically and mentally.

By adopting chair yoga as part of your daily routine, you will become more aware of the present moment, which will result in better focus and emotional stability.

You will establish a healthier relationship with the food you consume, and you will become more aware of the taste, smell, and sensations that food creates in your body. Once you start eating mindfully, you will need far fewer portions during meals.

You will no longer overeat; you will not consume food to suppress your emotions.

This chapter will show you why establishing a regular chair yoga practice is essential to your existence, physically and mentally.

THE CONECTION OF STRESS TO AGING, HEALTH, AND WEIGHT LOSS

If you are exposed to stress for most of the day, it can create or worsen:

- Hormonal imbalance
- Cognitive decline
- Accelerated cell aging
- Cardiovascular problems
- Compromised immune system

- Digestive problems
- Metabolic issues
- Emotional overeating

Hormonal imbalance: If you are exposed to stress most of the day, it will lead to the release of the hormone cortisol. It certainly won't be good for your body because elevated levels of this hormone generally lead to stronger inflammatory processes.

Stronger inflammatory processes have a bad effect on your overall health and, therefore, on the aging process.

***

FREE GIFT #4: E-BOOK "ANTI-INFLAMMATORY DIET FOR SENIORS"

Elevate your health and accelerate your weight loss journey with a diet plan focused on reducing inflammation and shedding excess pounds. This e-book complements the physical benefits of chair yoga exercises by addressing inflammation, a common cause of weight gain and discomfort.

To get your copy, visit **bit.ly/YogaBonuses**

You can also scan the QR code with your phone camera if you prefer not to type. It's absolutely free.

I hope this helps you achieve your health and weight loss goals every day.

***

Cognitive decline: Cognitive decline (the brain aging process) can occur because of chronic stress. Chronic stress is one of the main factors that cause neurodegenerative diseases.

Accelerated cellular aging: The length of your telomeres can shorten due to chronic stress, causing your cells to age faster. This results in premature biological aging.

What are telomeres?

Telomeres are vital to the preservation of information in your genome. Located at both ends of each chromosome, they are unique DNA protein structures whose main role is to protect the genome from nucleolytic degradation.

Cardiovascular problems: If you are constantly exposed to stress, it generally leads to high blood pressure and increases the risk of various heart diseases and other cardiovascular disorders.

Compromised immune system: The more you are exposed to stress, the more your immune system weakens. Your body becomes more susceptible to diseases and infections.

Digestive problems: Chronic stress can lead to poorer absorption of nutrients and thus make the digestive process more difficult and affect weight control.

Metabolic Issues: Metabolic balance can be disturbed in situations where there is an imbalance of hormones in your body. Due to hormonal imbalance, metabolism no longer functions properly, causing an increase in body weight or severe weight loss.

Emotional overeating: When you are under stress, you often resort to emotional eating. We are talking about food that contains a high level of sugar and fat. In the short run, you will be stress-free; however, in the long run, emotional overeating leads to excessive weight gain.

WHAT IS STRESS, AND HOW DOES IT ARISE?

To attain good health, slow down the aging process, and achieve an ideal body weight, it is very important to understand what stress is, how it arises, and how you can control it.

Stress is your body's natural response to threats or challenges.

Stress is technically good because it increases concentration and focus. You are more aware of the present moment because your body is in "fight or flight" mode.

Stress triggers various physiological and psychological reactions within your body, leading to the mobilization of resources to address the threat or challenge.

However, the longer your body is exposed to stress, the more damaging it becomes.

How do you control stress?

To gain control over stressful situations, it is very important to practice some of the following:

- Breathing techniques
- Regular exercise
- Mindfulness and meditation
- Mindful eating
- Positive thinking
- Enough sleep
- Establish a healthy lifestyle
- Good time management
- Learn to say **NO**
- Indulge in relaxing activities

Breathing techniques: By applying the breathing techniques explained in this book, you will be able to relax your nervous system and strengthen your nerves.

If you want to control stress in the right way, I advise you to regularly practice belly breathing and sound S breathing.

With these breathing techniques, you'll relax your nervous system and body muscles.

Regular exercise: When you exercise regularly, you release endorphins, a hormone that positively affects your mood.

This is why it is important to establish a daily chair yoga practice.

REGULAR CHAIR YOGA PRACTICE = SECRETION OF ENDORPHINS = STRESS CONTROL

Mindfulness and meditation: Chair yoga is a mindfulness activity, as during practice you breathe consciously, improving your focus and concentration.

You also become mindful when you do one thing at a time; forget about multitasking.

Another mindfulness activity is taking a walk, preferably alone in nature or silently with your partner. This is known as a meditative walk, which features silence, the only sounds coming from your breathing and nature.

Of course, you can also practice meditation at home.

A very simple meditation can be practiced on the chair you use during chair yoga. Just close your eyes, straighten your back, bend your chin slightly towards your sternum, and focus your attention on each inhale and exhale.

Focus on the expansion of the abdomen, the chest, and the lifting of the tops of the lungs.

Try to make each exhalation twice as long as your inhalation.

In the beginning, it is okay for you to meditate for one minute (one or two weeks).

The most important thing is that you feel comfortable during meditation, and you don't feel it as something imposed on you.

Over time, you can increase the number of minutes of meditation.

There is no exact number of minutes for which meditation can be said to be the most useful.

For some people, only a few minutes are enough; for others, it takes tens of minutes or more.

Listen to your body!

Mindful eating: If you haven't practiced mindful eating before, maybe this is the right time to start.

What is mindful eating?

Mindful eating means always expressing gratitude for the food before you. Thank whoever you want; this is not a religious concept; thank the chef who prepared your meal if you are in a restaurant or have ordered takeout (you don't have to say thank you out loud; it's perfectly okay to silently express gratitude). Through the act of gratitude, you raise the overall positive frequency of your body and become more aware of the meal in front of you.

During mindful eating, try to eat in silence without any distractions (turn off the TV, try not to talk during the meal, especially not while you have food in your mouth).

If you eat this way, you will:

- Become aware of your every bite
- Swallow sufficiently chewed food, and you will not swallow it unconsciously
- Eat at the right speed; you won't swallow too much air (this happens when you eat unconsciously or too fast)
- Feel full with much smaller portions

Food is very important for the proper functioning of your body. That is why the food you eat and the way you eat is important.

If you haven't included **super foods** in your menu, maybe it's time to start consuming them.

Super foods are foods that have a great effect on your body because of their essential mineral content.

Below is a list of super foods that I regularly consume:

- Dark leafy greens
- Green tea
- Legumes
- Eggs
- Berries
- Seeds
- Nuts
- Garlic
- Kefir
- Ginger

- Olive oil
- Salmon
- Curcumin
- Sweet potato
- Avocado
- Seaweed
- Mushrooms

If you want to achieve your ideal body weight, please start your mindful eating practice. If you would like to learn more about mindful eating – check out our book on this subject.

****

FREE GIFT #5: E-BOOK "MINDFUL EATING"

Achieve your ideal body weight with mindful eating. Our e-book, "Mindful Eating: Develop a Better Relationship with Food through Mindfulness," offers essential tips to overcome eating disorders, enjoy healthy weight loss, and improve your relationship with food.

Get your copy at **bit.ly/YogaBonuses** or scan the QR code. It's absolutely free.

I hope this e-book helps you on your journey to better health.

****

This book is packed with essential tips and tricks about how you can begin changing your diet for the better, develop a better relationship with food through mindfulness and subsequently improve your life.

Positive thinking: Try not to let negative thoughts fill your mind. Replace them with positive thoughts.

One of the easiest ways to incorporate this into your daily practice is through positive affirmations.

It is also important to be aware of situations you cannot change and accept them. There's no need to get upset about those situations, especially since you can't change them.

You should focus on things and situations in your control. By investing energy in such things, you will positively change your thought process.

Get enough sleep: It is very important to create a healthy bedtime routine (cleaning your face, teeth, evening bath, meditation, etc.).

Try to always go to bed at the same time.

Pay attention to the quality of your mattress and pillow. The average life of a mattress is about 10 years, and that of pillows is about 3 years. If you feel that you are no longer comfortable in bed, it may be the right time to think about changing your mattress and pillows.

Good time management: Organize your tasks daily and weekly. Prioritize them according to importance. Always do the most important tasks first.

If some tasks seem overwhelming, divide them into smaller, more manageable chunks.

Learn to say NO: Do not accept more obligations or tasks imposed on you by other people that don't align with your capabilities and current aspirations.

Learn to say no; otherwise, you will be overwhelmed by emotions. The accumulation of emotions can lead to weight gain. This is why it is important to learn to say NO.

Indulge in relaxing activities: Start spending more time doing activities that bring you joy and happiness. If you have a hobby or several hobbies, dedicate yourself to them.

Spend more time in nature, listen to relaxing music, and engage in activities that involve working with your hands (gardening, sculpting, drawing, cooking, etc.).

In this chapter, you learned the definition of stress and how it impacts aging, health, and weight.

You also learned how to control the stress you are exposed to. By applying the mentioned techniques, you will resolve your stress, and when you get stress under control, it will impact your body and weight loss.

CONCLUSION

Chair yoga goes beyond exercise. The combination of mindful movement, conscious breathing, and a strong commitment to good health pave the way for change.

Chair yoga is a transformative practice that rethinks the relationship between the mind, body, and spirit. It is more than just a series of poses.

Every pose, every breath, and every mindful moment combined make chair yoga a wonderful practice for losing weight.

Chair yoga for weight loss is a process rather than a goal, and it requires embracing yourself as much as losing weight.

Chair yoga has various advantages for people of all ages, especially those with restricted mobility or physical problems.

It improves total physical function by increasing flexibility, strength, and balance.

Furthermore, the practice involves mindfulness and deep breathing, which contribute to stress reduction, enhanced mental focus, and relaxation, making it a comprehensive approach to well-being.

Furthermore, chair yoga is easily customizable to individual needs, allowing participants to work at their own pace and grow at their own pace as they feel comfortable.

The practice can also help relieve joint pain and stiffness, making it appropriate for people suffering from arthritis or other musculoskeletal ailments. Chair yoga, being a low-impact workout, is a handy and accessible choice for people of all abilities, and fosters a good attitude toward regular physical activity.

To enjoy the process, please follow the detailed instructions within the book and adhere to the guidelines provided.

And, of course, stay motivated!

WOULD YOU DO ME A FOVOR?

Now that you've mastered the art of Chair Yoga, it's time to share your newfound knowledge and guide other seniors on their journey to a more active, pain-free life.

By sharing your honest opinion of this book on Amazon, you can point other seniors in the direction of the same valuable guidance you've found. Your review is more than just a few words; it's a beacon of hope for others seeking to regain their youthfulness and vitality.

Thank you for your contribution. The movement towards better health and flexibility for seniors is fueled by the wisdom we share – and your review plays a crucial role in this mission.

To leave your review on Amazon go to this link:

amzn.to/42eZEud

Or scan QR code with your camera:

Your voice matters. By leaving a review, you're not just helping others discover this book; you're becoming part of a larger story. A story where every senior has the chance to feel younger, more agile, and enjoy life to its fullest.

Together, we're keeping the spirit of youthful living alive. Your review is a powerful tool in this journey, and I am deeply grateful for your support.

Thank you for being a part of this incredible community. Let's continue to inspire and uplift each other, one stretch at a time.

We strongly believe that there are a thousand ways to improve your life and health. However, there is no single recipe suitable for everyone how to do that.

We think that the best way to receive your goals is the one you can stick to and our writers will do their best to provide simple, easy to follow, step by step and realistic instructions how to do that.

To discover our best books go to link:

amzn.to/40B5KmZ

Or scan QR code with your camera:

REFERENCES

1. Vive Health. Feb 2, (2020, February 2). Seated Jumping Jacks Chair Exercise. Video. YouTube.
https://www.youtube.com/watch?v=zKZOVD30vK0

2. Vive Health. Feb 2, (2020, February 2). Seated Toe Tap Exercise. Video. YouTube.
https://www.youtube.com/watch?v=T4uJ4DXQy04

3. Sworkit Health. (n.d.) *How to do knee to chest.*
https://sworkit.com/exercise/knee-to-chest.

4. Reneu Health. (2020, March 31). *You May Wanna Sit Down for This...* https://www.reneu-health.com/post/you-may-wanna-sit-down-for-this?fbclid=IwAR1XKfhZXJ8WsSYkaA_j11mvK3ZZ0elFn1CCt0KaFkz26aZtngIJfTVnJ3Q

5. Tummee. (n.d.) *Seated Chair One Hand Behind Head Elbow Knee Flow.* https://www.tummee.com/yoga-poses/seated-chair-one-hand-behind-head-elbow-knee-flow

6. WorkoutLabs. (n.d.) *Seated cat cow.*
https://workoutlabs.com/exercise-guide/seated-cat-cow/

7. Sondhi Dutt, S. (2016, February 16). *5 Chair Yoga Poses You Can Do Anywhere.*
https://yogawithsapna.com/5-chair-yoga-poses/

8. Tummee. (n.d.) *Alternate Shoulder Shrugs Close Up.*
https://www.tummee.com/yoga-poses/alternate-shoulder-shrugs-close-up

9. Arana, J. (2023, September 26). *How to Tone Legs While Sitting.*
https://www.wikihow.com/Tone-Legs-While-Sitting

10. Stafford, T. (2023, August 26). *How to Do Reverse Crunches.*
https://www.wikihow.com/Do-Reverse-Crunches

11. Tummee. (n.d.) *Knee Head Down Chair.*
https://www.tummee.com/yoga-poses/knee-head-down-chair

12. Age Bold. (2020, February 12). Lace up your sneakers and come exercise with us for Age Bold's #MoveOfTheDay! Today we're working with seated mountain climbers. Facebook.
https://www.facebook.com/watch/?v=1752475737769686

13. Ankrom, S. (2023, January 27). *9 Breathing Exercises to Relieve Anxiety.*
https://www.verywellmind.com/abdominal-breathing-2584115

14. National Library of Medicine. (2020, July 7). *The Link between Chronic Stress and Accelerated Aging.*
https://www.ncbi.nlm.nih.gov/pmc/articles/PMC7400286/

15. Shammas, M. (2020, July 7). *Telomeres, lifestyle, cancer, and aging.*
https://www.ncbi.nlm.nih.gov/pmc/articles/PMC3370421/

16. Felson, S. (2023, September 12). *Ways to manage stress.*
https://www.webmd.com/balance/stress-management/stress-management

17. Ajmera, R. (2021, February 22). *16 Superfoods That Are Worthy of the Title.*
https://www.healthline.com/nutrition/14-healthiest-vegetables-on-earth#TOC_TITLE_HDR_8

Made in the USA
Monee, IL
12 July 2025